P

Now Everyone Will Know

"I first met Maggie Kneip when she was nine months pregnant with her second child. Less than a year later, her husband, John, would die of AIDS. In the wake of this unspeakable trauma, I watched Maggie bravely, tirelessly rebuild her life and raise two extraordinary kids. Familiar as I was with her story, nothing prepared me for the transcendent power of *Now Everyone Will Know*. Maggie's unflinchingly honest memoir of loss, grief, and ultimately triumphant self-discovery is a book for anyone affected by the plague of AIDS, anyone who has struggled to process grief and make sense of the bewildering randomness of life and death."

—**Tony Goldwyn,** actor and director

"This is a book I just inhaled. I could not put it down. Maggie Kneip is a courageous and beautiful writer, willing to bare all the painful chapters in her life. There is something universal in her story. It will resonate with every woman who has something to hide—and that is most of us, myself included."

—**Magee Hickey,** news reporter, WPIX-TV New York

"Maggie Kneip was one of this country's hidden women: an AIDS widow who kept her husband's deadly secret for more than two decades to protect her children from stigma. Now she opens up for the first time in this stunning, beautifully written and important book. *Now Everyone Will Know* is a heartbreaking yet ultimately triumphant tale of love, loss, betrayal—and redemption."

—**Joanne Lipman,** journalist, editor, and co-author of *Strings Attached*

"*Now Everyone Will Know* is by turns surprising, heartbreaking, inspiring, and funny. Maggie Kneip's story of love, loss, and betrayal will move you, and it will haunt you. Like Isabel Gillies and Marco Roth, Kneip writes of the secrets families keep, and the wreckage such secrets can cause. This is an important book, not just because it's a fascinating memoir, but because it's a powerful historical document about the devastating effects of the AIDS crisis and a moving meditation on the wages of love."

—**Melissa Kirsch,** author of *The Girl's Guide to Absolutely Everything*

"I helped take care of John Andrew, my brilliant boss at *The Wall Street Journal*, at the dawn of the AIDS epidemic, a barely remembered moment marked by fear and stigma and certain death. John died with extraordinary speed, leaving most unsaid. Now close to three decades later, his widow, Maggie Kneip, has recaptured John's unique voice, while also chronicling, with honesty and courage, her struggle to accept the enduring mystery at the core of their relationship. A meditation on loss, forgiveness, and the ties that bind, *Now Everyone Will Know* is indelible."

—**Alix M. Freedman,** journalist

"Maggie Kneip has gathered the exquisite details of her heartbreaking journey like lilies from a field, wrapped them in words of brutal honesty, and delivered a debut memoir that serves up laughter and deep-belly sorrow in equal measure. To render the unspeakable in such a way that provides a necessary healing for not only the writer but readers as well is a gift. *Now Everyone Will Know* tells a new story of the ones often left out of the tale of the AIDS epidemic—the ones left behind."

—**Katori Hall**, actress, journalist, playwright, and 2010 Olivier Award winner for Broadway's *The Mountaintop*

Now
Everyone
Will Know

Now Everyone Will Know

THE PERFECT HUSBAND, HIS SHATTERING SECRET, MY REDISCOVERED LIFE

{A MEMOIR}

MAGGIE KNEIP

FOREWORD BY LAURA LANDRO
AFTERWORD BY DR. DALE ATKINS

GARDEN STREET BOOKS / NEW YORK

GARDEN STREET BOOKS

www.gardenstreetbooks.com

Library of Congress Control Number: 2015952901
ISBN 978-0-692-53781-7
Printed in the United States of America
Art direction by JENNIFER K. BEAL DAVIS
Cover design by JENNIFER K. BEAL DAVIS
Interior layout by BRETT MILLER
Cover illustrations designed by Freepik

First Edition

1 3 5 7 9 10 8 6 4 2

For anyone having to hold back the truth

"I think I've created memories. Or maybe this is real. It's a memory I have of him leaving our apartment in Hoboken, me asking him where he was going, and someone telling me he was going to heaven. I was so little, though. It must have been a dream."

—CAROLINE ANDREW

Foreword

I first met John Andrew in the late 1980s when I was covering the media and entertainment industry for *The Wall Street Journal*, and he was a top reporter on the financial markets beat. Hardly your typical journalist, he looked more like the investment bankers and traders he wrote about, with his perfect white shirts and well-tailored suits. He had a sharp grasp of the machinations of the stock market and corporate finance; writing for our popular "Heard on the Street" column, he even made subjects like property-casualty insurance shares sound intriguing. One day he'd be writing about the thrift industry, the next about toy stocks.

Our beats crossed when the deals began to heat up in my industry, and we collaborated on stories about the frenzy beginning to grip broadcasting, cable, and entertainment companies. In 1987, we shared a byline in a major story about the battle between Warner Communications and its largest shareholder,

Chris-Craft, which would ultimately end in the merger of Time Inc. and Warner. It was one of the major business sagas of that era, and it would consume much of our time for months. I was sourced on the personalities and the drama, but it was John who brought the deep knowledge of the financial issues at stake—the lifeblood for our readers.

John's star was on the rise, and he was soon named the editor of our team of about a dozen reporters, which spanned not only media but marketing, advertising, publishing, food, alcohol, tobacco, and retailing. He had a glass-walled office that looked out over our patch of cubicles in the *Journal*'s World Financial Center offices, and was usually in there smoking away—which you could do in those days—and working his magic on our (often very) raw copy.

I usually got a little overexcited when news broke, especially when I had a scoop, and would rush into his office after I'd filed a story to deal with his questions. Sometimes I was nervous we'd miss the deadline as he sat there puffing on his cigarette and crafting the story more artfully, making sure I'd bulletproofed the facts. He'd stare at his screen and fiddle with the lead to make it more compelling while I sat there practically hyperventilating, but he always wrapped it up and pushed the button to zap the story to the news desk right under the wire.

More times than I can count, one particular executive would call the next day with a complaint about something I'd written, and when I couldn't get him off the phone I'd transfer the call to John, then peek into his office to watch him rolling his eyes, holding the phone slightly away from his ear, and calming the guy down. He was the perfect boss in a way: he didn't drive you crazy, trusted you to do your work, and helped immeasurably to make you a better reporter and writer.

When I met John's wife, Maggie, I was duly impressed; this buttoned-up, perfect Ivy League WASP had married a creative and artsy, yet down-to-earth and direct, "nice Jewish girl." Their daughter, Caroline, was a toddler and their son, Daniel, just an infant, and both were Gerber-baby adorable. They were living a great life in a gentrified yet still hip Hoboken neighborhood and seemed like the perfect young family, with a bright future together.

But suddenly, one day, John wasn't at work. And before long, a story more devastating than any of us could imagine began to unfold. Maggie went overnight from a happy young mother raising her children with a loving husband to a woman struck by an unexpected and unimaginable tragedy. The strength she found from within to bring herself and her children through that time would prove to be their salvation, but the journey itself was a nightmare that most of us were powerless to help with in those early days, let alone understand.

To see where they have all come to today, despite such a profound trauma, is to appreciate the power of love, resilience, and determination, which Maggie has in abundance. And the world has come a long way, too: though eternal vigilance will be necessary, a virulent disease has been brought under control, and a generation of activism has removed the stigma and fear that once surrounded it. But it has also become easier to forget what happened at the beginning, when it wasn't like that at all, and there was nowhere to turn for help or understanding.

There are countless stories about the many men who lost

their lives to that plague, but there is much left unsaid about the families some left behind. This is one of those stories, and it needs to be told.

LAURA LANDRO
New York, New York
September 2015

Preface

The day my daughter graduated from Brown University, she asked me a surprising question. Light rain fell from the Providence skies that Sunday in May 2009. Caroline's class had walked through the historic Van Wickle Gates behind alumni of the class of 1976, of which her deceased father was a member.

"Didn't you think today was sad?" she asked from beneath the shadow of her mortarboard. "I looked at the class of '76, and thought, where's Dad? Why isn't he here?"

The question had loomed over us long before Caroline's time at Brown, and I was determined not to let it ruin her proud, happy day. But there was no denying it was sad. Caroline was three when her father died in 1991. Her younger brother, Dan, who was born in 1990, never knew his father at all. In all the intervening years, we had barely spoken of him.

Now she was asking about him. "Where's Dad?" As a way of answering this question, and of perhaps coming to terms with what had happened to him, and to us, this was something I needed to change.

It was finally time to talk about John.

Magski,

You are the original spark of life. I know I don't talk much, but this year has been the happiest of my life. I love you very much.

Johnski

One

I could have used someone as steady, strong, and smart as John Andrew in my life as early as second grade, when, in the comments section of my report card, my teacher wrote, "Margaret is very nervous. How can we get her to relax?" It was true; I was always frenetic, reaching, panicked about making mistakes or not being the best. My anxiety was in full swing well before the morning bell sounded, having protected my older brother, Bill, on our long walk to school, hurrying him past the lurking bullies. Why couldn't my parents see what I did? How different he was? How slow.

Bill was just one of many disabled kids left to fall through the cracks back then, and I was the sibling anointed to make it all better. Not just better, nigh on perfect. "Reach for the stars!" my mother advised from beneath her Jackie Kennedyesque pillbox hat.

My mother, Carolyn Zuckerman Kneip, was a true believer in self-improvement. Sprung from the poverty-stricken,

Yiddishkeit streets of Brooklyn, she dreamed of Camelot. Her favorite oft-told childhood anecdote—one of very few she stingily shared—was about her older brother, Joe, the only one of her three brothers she ever mentioned. Instead of being a *balagula* (Yiddish for "wagon driver") like the others, Joe was an attorney, educated and refined. "One day, when I was about fifteen," she'd say, her intense brown eyes widening, "Joe grabbed the romance magazine right out of my hands and *replaced it with Dostoyevsky!*"

My mother credited this single act for nothing less than saving her life, teaching her that there was a world far beyond Brooklyn for the yearning. At the University of Pennsylvania, where she worked as a secretary, she was inspired by the celebrated Professor Martin Seligman, who famously espoused the theory of "authentic happiness." To fervent disciples like my mother, anything was possible and within reach (so long as she didn't take a hard look at her son).

There aren't any pictures of my mother until she was in her early thirties, when she met my father, Arthur Kneip, a Jew from Virginia who wore Brooks Brothers suits, graduated from a classy college, and had the means for a camera.

My father was raised in a ramshackle Tidewater Virginia house overflowing with cousins by his soft-spoken, widowed mother on a hopeful diet of Old Testament sound bites and penny-saver proverbs. Though short and stocky, he stood tall as the man in the family, working in the local shipyards from a young age to help support her and a younger sister. By the time he met my mother, he'd risen far above poverty, donning the corporate cufflinks of a national sales manager in what was then a booming Detroit, hawking industrial electrical products and managing to survive three corporate takeovers.

My dad was a survivor, and years later, after duking it out all day with his accounts, he'd come home to the dinner table with his gloves still on, often sending a verbal jab our way. The steaming lasagna would have barely cooled before he'd counsel, "Get thinner if you want the boys to like you," as he reached for more bread. "And be a lady. Try not to be so funny all the time. Men don't like women who are fat and funny."

I'd slam down my fork, eyes stinging. It wasn't my fault I was a hair chunkier than my girlfriends. I was built like him, though he was apparently blind to this genetic connection. True, I was pretty—blond and blue-eyed, a perfect *shana maidela* ("beautiful maiden") to everyone's grandmother—but this wasn't a Polish shtetl, it was the Motown sixties, when Diana Ross and waiflike Twiggy reigned supreme. As for my sense of humor, if I could make you laugh I was darn well going to do it—or anything else necessary to deflect comments about my size or my tag-along brother, to whom my father would turn next, badgering Bill for "hanging back" and having "no drive."

My mother skillfully sidestepped this suppertime fracas by introducing conversational topics of no relevance. "Do you know about the fascinating author Primo Levi?" she'd ask.

Any parenting advice came from Dr. Haim Ginott on the *Today* show, to whom they listened with half an ear during breakfast. It was a different time.

I tried to fulfill both my mother's star-seeking aspirations and my father's ideal of femininity by becoming a dancer. I loved the feeling of soaring far above it all, a perfect plié setting things right. But my body, of course, was all wrong, and no amount of swimming laps or squat thrusting, no amount of dolefully refusing ice cream or pizza, could change it.

In college, I took up residence in the campus dance studio, considering nothing else for a career. But after moving to New York City upon graduation and finding myself taking more drink orders than curtain calls, I felt my chance for stardom begin to dim. I wondered if I could find bright lights in someone else instead—a man, for example. Jeff was an elegant, black, Ivy-educated banker and I fell for him, fast. But after nearly three years together, when he was accepted to Harvard Business School and the question of marriage came up, we let the strident disapproval of our parents, not to mention society at large, break us apart.

It was a different time.

Twenty-seven, heartbroken, convinced that I'd never find another man as luminous, I threw myself back into performing, this time in regional dinner theater and a flea-bitten dance company. When not onstage, I'd bunk up with college roommates in their Hell's Kitchen railroad apartment and moonlight as a singing waitress at a Bowery seafood shack, occasionally getting fixed up with someone's cousin. Then, one chilly spring night, I entered a Tribeca bar to meet a blind date whose beautiful red hair gave off an unmistakable glow.

When my high school friend set me up with John Andrew, a guy she'd known at Brown and at Harvard Business School, I expected a man with dandruff and a pocket protector. John's hair wasn't merely red; it was titian, a vibrant red named for the sixteenth-century Venetian painter. He was dressed stylishly yet whimsically, with a closely cut suit of beautiful fabric, imported loafers, chic horn-rimmed glasses, and an of-the-moment accessory: an orange Swatch watch. Beneath the clothes was, I could tell, a toned, strong, compact body.

Charmingly, John did most of the listening, and we stayed so long we closed the bar. Later, the image he cast in the streetlight—a voluminous navy wool overcoat he wore adorned with a red scarf—mesmerized me. Before we went our separate ways, he shoved me against the subway station's cold tiled wall and kissed me, hard. At first, I felt ambushed—bruised—and wanted to push him away, but then I became lost in it, and in him. I fairly swooned home.

Soon we were spending every free minute together. I loved everything about John: how he looked, his brownstone apartment tucked into a leafy Hoboken back street, and even more the eclectic book and record collection lining its floor-to-ceiling shelves. There were Goethe (in German), Fielding, Bellow, and Faulkner. There was hip pulp crime fiction by someone named Jim Thompson. He owned a treasure trove of albums: Roy Orbison, Marianne Faithfull, the Talking Heads, the Stones, Tom Waits.

There was a quiet power about John, an *über*-competence in all things. He was unfailingly meticulous, from his dress to his table manners, to what he said, to what he wrote and edited for *The Wall Street Journal*. His clever front-page articles ranged from the profile of a quirky California couple who called themselves "the apostles of life extension" to crack investigative reporting on financial fraud. John was a master of dispensing just enough information to make a story sing. When his reporters panicked on deadline, he'd sweep in at the last moment, cigarette dangling, and type in just the right closing lines with minutes to spare. Word was, the bigger the crisis, the calmer John got. His talented group of reporters revered him for his relaxed assuredness and deft touch in editing their stories.

Best of all, John valued everything in me that my father had diminished. As someone who tended toward prolonged periods of silence, he relished my talent for piping up to fill a conversational gap. "You're the original spark of life," he'd say, beaming. For him, I "lit up a room!"

Sometimes I'd become ruffled by John's silences, wondering just what it was he wasn't sharing. He always apologized, often winsomely. Once, after a tiff about his laconic nature, he crafted a *mea culpa* set to the tune of Sam Cooke's "Wonderful World" that read: "I got an 'A' in biology, but got an 'F' in talking-ology. Still, I know that I love you, and I have a wonderful time with you!" Winsome creativity flowed from his every pore.

It was hard to stay angry with John. Almost every day, I awoke to a greeting card or note scribbled with "I wuv you!" or "To my sexy, funny, pretty, smart, charming (in any order you want), Magski." When, shortly after we met, I followed John's suggestion to drop my theatrical aspirations and "get a real job" by taking a position in public relations, he sent a giant telegram to my new office reading, "Here's to a transcendent transition, baby. Love, Johnski." The decision became infinitely more palatable.

From the very first minute of our very first meeting, I could feel John's heat. He had a bit of the Clark Kent thing about him: take off the glasses, open the shirt, and... I loved guys like that. Don't most women? Eventually, we adopted a summer Sunday routine of waking up before dawn, grabbing coffee and bagels, and speeding out to Long Island's Jones Beach, where he would lead me back to the tall beach grass and push me down to the sand. Ignoring my cries from an occasional broken shell or stone, he'd slip his hand under the elastic of my bathing suit bottom and devilishly finger me. Ummm. That was the essence of him, so much impact with so little effort, be it talking—or foreplay. Soon he'd begin thrusting in that powerful, sinewy way he had. By then, the sun was rising and people were arriving with their kids and coolers, kicking up sand around us. I'd cry, "John! What if they see us?" and he'd cover my mouth and bear down. I'd arch up and then, well, who cared about anything, really?

John was, most assuredly, a star. After six months of dating and a year of living together, he took me to dinner at the Odeon, a restaurant we loved in Tribeca, and asked me to marry him. I was elated, and so were my parents. John possessed precisely the qualities their own son lacked, including God-given talent. It didn't matter one whit that he wasn't Jewish.

About ten weeks before our wedding, my mother sent a draft of our wedding invitation to John (not me) for his approval, accompanied by the following note:

Dear John,

I suppose there is no need to repeat all the superlatives thrown into Maggie's ears this morning when we spoke, but it rarely hurts to hurl a few compliments your way once again... You are a lucky pair and we are very pleased. Bill is out now at a party of sorts but intends to let you know how grateful he is you made such an effort to fix his bike... Thanks, John.

About the decorating ideas we discussed—I haven't had time to see the Home Furnishings section in the Times *today (the section has some good hints I think)… I love your apartment—in fact, so does Arthur… Please show the enclosed to Maggie so that I may be able to correct whatever you think should be changed and go ahead with the order. Can't think of anything else to say.*
—C.K.

John could discuss invitations and living room design with my mother, give my father bragging rights, and fix my brother's bike. I'd picked the perfect man for everyone.

Less enthused about our match—and my Jewish background—was John's father, Merle, who refused to attend our wedding. Merle didn't much like John's career choice of journalism, either. Raised poor in Nebraska yet having earned a doctorate from MIT, he expected nothing less from either of his sons than Nobel Prizes and big paychecks. His elder son, Robert, had risen to the occasion, earning a PhD in economics and serving as the CFO of an investment bank, but John, a mere newspaper editor—a "copy processor," as Merle called it—had fatally missed the mark.

Nonetheless, on August 31, 1986, in a glass-enclosed Chelsea loft infused with summer sunlight, John and I were married. He stamped on the glass, we were pronounced husband and wife, and Paul Simon's "Graceland," that year's chart topper, rang out as our recessional. For me, the song symbolized the consummate state of grace I'd attained by marrying my smart, seamless John; its exuberant sounds of zydeco, rock, and South African *a capella* harmonies conveyed my unbridled joy.

One year later, our beautiful daughter, Caroline, was born. Our ride to the hospital was pure Keystone Kops with a dash of Laurel and Hardy: "Ohmigod, my water broke! Ohmigod, get the bag, no, wait, you get the car, I'll get the bag. Wait, the keys—I thought *you* had the keys? Ohmigod, get some towels, this water is gushing... Get the car. *Get the car!*"

John and his dented Datsun sped me and my smelly towels through the Lincoln Tunnel to Mount Sinai Hospital, where for twenty-one hours I labored with him hovering close, mopping my brow and cracking jokes while exhaling me through our Lamaze regimen. Finally, I batted him away, bellowing, "Get the drug guy!"

When it was all over, after the last seismic push that sent our beautiful daughter into the world, I felt a gentle, warm washcloth in my battered nether region: John, tenderly cleaning me up. "I love you, baby," he whispered. "You're going to be a wonderful mother."

After the birth of our daughter, John and I cozily cocooned in Hoboken. Things felt so blemishless, we reminded ourselves of the Bohemian-bourgeois yuppies Hope and Michael on our favorite TV show, *Thirtysomething*. Hoboken back then was like Brooklyn today, its streets lined with cafés and corner bars, vibrant with journalists, authors, actors, filmmakers, and musicians. I swam laps next to Tony Goldwyn, the gorgeous young star of the hit movie *Ghost*; shared a babysitter with Oscar-winning actor Chris Cooper; and rode the bus with Pulitzer Prize–winner Anna Quindlen, then author of a weekly *New York Times* column called "Life in the 30s." Indie filmmaker John Sayles shot hoops at our local YMCA, while the co-creator of *Hair*, James Rado, lived just down the street. Catty-corner from our condo was the now-legendary Maxwell's, headlining the best in punk and indie rock music. Italian widows, draped head-to-toe in black, peppered the pavement and the air smelled enticingly of frying dough and coffee grinding at the Maxwell House factory. Across the filthy yet glinting Hudson stood Manhattan in all its glory. Where better to be thirty-something in 1990?

Each weekday morning after John left for work, I'd make a mad dash for the Y to join "my girls"—a posse of fitness-freak moms with whom I did just about everything—for a five-mile run while our babies rolled around its child-care center. We reveled in our daily locker room banter about TV and movies, our petty marital spats and whiny kids, our preferences in disposable diaper brands. Then we'd eagerly burst through the Y's heavy double doors and prance like proud Lipizzaners, evenly spaced, knees high, onto a sweep of road in Hoboken on the banks of the Hudson known as Frank Sinatra Drive. We loved running and, even more, running with each other.

Come Friday night, our husbands would loosen their ties, mix up intoxicating pitchers, and fire up the grill. John, having replaced his Brioni suit with a perfectly broken-in pair of jeans and lovingly preserved blue t-shirt from college, was our chef, cooking the burgers impeccably. After dinner we'd pool our money and send someone out for a couple decent bottles of Merlot, then sit around the grill's dying embers, babies dozing on our laps, drinking and talking long into the night. John could always be counted on to spark discourse and elicit laughs with one or two well-timed remarks. I preened. So smart, my husband! My own boozy contributions to the conversation had a tendency to ramble on; when they did, I would sense even in the dark John's eyes rolling in semi-feigned exasperation. It was the same treatment his reporters joked about at cocktail parties. John always knew when we'd said too much.

Later, I'd put our daughter to bed and climb into ours. "I don't know what I'd do without you," I'd whisper, nestling into my husband's warm, rock-solid form.

On our second wedding anniversary, six months after Caroline was born, John gave me gorgeous Tiffany earrings with a card reading:

Dear Maggie,
No gift can express my love for you. But I like little presents, none-theless. Now we are three. We fight sometimes and we wish we had more money, but in truth I think we will look back on this as one of the best times of our lives. You are still, as always, the original spark of life, my sexy lover, and my best friend.
Love you always, Johnski

The following fall, things started to change. We were delighted when we found out I was pregnant again, and over the moon when the *Journal* picked John to oversee the launch of a historic third section of the paper. But during the ensuing months, as my girth swelled and our sweet daughter entered her "terrible twos," he started coming home later and later, his eyes tired and red. Even his hands were red, or rather, covered by an angry red rash—the doctor said it was psoriasis, attributable to stress. Stress was apparently also behind John's exhaustion, frequent coughs, and intestinal turbulence. He began to see a psychiatrist to manage it all.

All through that winter, as John's mood darkened, I kept a stiff upper lip. I had to, minding a small child while pregnant with another. If I voiced concern, John would rebut it with, "It's nothing. I'm tired. I could use a break, that's all. " Sometimes he would add, "And I'm worried about money," propelling me to solicit freelance writing assignments and choreography jobs. I was glad to do it; anything to relieve his mounting stress, which, if it continued, would kill us both.

One Saturday in late June, our son announced himself with sharp contractions. This time around, John and I left for the hospital in an orderly fashion, the silence of our drive broken only by my occasional whimper. At the hospital, the obstetrician pronounced me "just about there"—an hour or so from labor, in fact—whereupon John rose from his bedside chair and announced, "I'm just heading out for a quick bite."

The doctor and I shot each other a glance.

"Now?" I asked.

"I'm hungry," he said. "I'll be back in time." He patted my hand and left.

A sharp pain shot through my abdomen. The hell with his goddamn burger and fries, I was having a baby! No—not *a* baby—*his* baby! The doctor mumbled something about checking on another patient and left me with the nurses.

As usual, John's timing was perfect. He made it back just in time to witness the birth of his son, Daniel, who tipped the scales at nearly eleven pounds. A few minutes after labor, as the doctor handed our son to me, I realized that John had disappeared once again. "I had a call from work," he later explained.

During the two weeks John was on paternity leave, he could

barely get up off the couch. You'd have thought he was the one who'd just given birth to a size XL baby boy. Something had to be done to alleviate my beleaguered husband's debilitating stress. His birthday, during his first week back at work, was the perfect opportunity for a relaxing, intimate dinner at his favorite Greenwich Village bistro.

It would be just what we both needed.

Dear Maggie,

You don't have a house yet but Toodie and I will get you one soon. Love you always,
John and CAROLINE!

P.S. Make way for buttons (Toodie #2)!

Two

If a single day can change a life forever, July 10, 1990, my husband's thirty-sixth birthday, changed mine.

John met me at the restaurant after work, his hair damp with sweat. We made small talk while our waiter delivered ice-cold drinks. I had a white-wine spritzer; John ordered a gin and tonic—a double—that he fairly inhaled. He burned through one cigarette after another. When had he become a chain smoker? It had to have been another high-stress day.

Our steaming platters of steak-frites arrived. He placed his cigarette carefully between his lips and inserted his tie between the buttons of his still-crisp oxford shirt to protect it from food stains, and began rhythmically tapping the sides of the salt and pepper dispensers. John approached food as he did deadline stories: with calm precision.

I took a bite of steak, regretfully pushing the frites to the side, my stubborn baby weight in mind. I gulped down another forkful—breastfeeding made me ravenous, and the meat was delicious. I glanced up to see how John was doing with his, but he hadn't touched it. Instead, he sat motionless, with a cigarette dangling from his lips and his chin in his hand. He suddenly picked up the ashtray, held it out to me, and said, "We need more ketchup."

A full bottle of Heinz was on the table right in front of him. Did he not see it?

He sat dumbfounded, holding the ashtray, with a straight face. I suppressed an urge to laugh. Picking up the hefty red bottle, I said, "That's not the ketchup, John. *This* is the ketchup."

From behind his chic glasses, John continued to stare at me with big, blue, confused eyes, taking the cigarette, now burned to a butt, out of his mouth and holding it in his hand. In the other, he dangled the ashtray. There were things he might have said next that would have made it okay—things like, "Wow! What am I saying? I'm exhausted," or, "No more drinking for me; I'm fried. Let's go home, can we?" But he said nothing. He just sat, unable to comprehend the difference between the ashtray and the ketchup bottle.

I didn't know what to do. I'd seen a lot of shifting moods in John recently, but befuddled wasn't one of them. No matter how worn out or down, he was always sharp, clear, fast—always the one with a "Plan B" or, if need be, "Plan C." *C'mon, John*, I prayed. *Snap out of it. Snap out of…whatever this is!*

He put down the cigarette butt, took off his glasses, calmly cleaned them using the napkin on his lap, placed them back on his impassive face, and resumed his blank stare. I don't know how many seconds—minutes?—passed before he slumped over the table, his head in his hands, and struggled to talk. "I can't," he started to say; then his sentence drifted off and he looked up at me, as if hoping I would help him fill in the words.

The room froze: the white-coated waiters; the sweating, hustling busboys; the clanking glasses and plates; the din of soft jazz from the trio in the corner. My stomach plummeted.

"Stay here," I said. "Don't move."

I somehow managed to gather change and make it over to the pay phone to dial John's brother, Robert, at his home in Connecticut. John and Robert were close and talked daily—sometimes more than once—from their respective offices. Robert's wife, Nancy, a Harvard-educated lawyer newly pregnant with their second child, answered the phone. When I told her what was happening, she met my panic with a bit of her own.

"Holy shit!" she exclaimed, and quickly summoned Robert.

Like John, Robert was brilliant and almost always calm, which he remained as I choked out a description of his brother's bizarre behavior. Concerned, he asked if I'd be able to get John home, then reminded me that he was scheduled to meet him for a birthday lunch the following day. "Why don't I see how he is then?" he offered. We agreed that I would call in the morning to let him know how his brother was and hung up. My heart sank. Robert and Nancy were all the way in Connecticut. What was I thinking, calling them? What could they do from there?

I made my way back to our table, where John appeared to be musing pleasantly, his chin resting in one hand, in the other a cigarette burning down to his knuckles. He gazed up at me as if to ask, "What's all the fuss about?" I felt his forehead. He was burning up! I signaled for the check, threw down a crumpled wad of cash, and eased him up and out of his seat. We made our way into the humid July air, where, fortunately, a cab was waiting.

We sped through the Holland Tunnel back to Hoboken. John slipped down low in the seat; I reached over periodically to check his forehead, as one does with sick children, harboring a fantasy that a sudden, inexplicable break in the fever would mercifully occur.

When we reached our building I paid the driver, eased John out of the cab, and half carried him up the three steep, winding flights to our condo, where blue metallic "It's a Boy!" balloons wafted overhead. I paid the babysitter and hustled her out. As soon as the door closed behind her, I rushed to the back bedroom, where John had limped, his ankle still swollen from a recent gym accident. He bent over from the edge of the bed, struggling to take off his shiny Bruno Magli loafers.

I helped him wriggle one foot free, then the other, then maneuvered him back onto the bed to remove his suit, shirt, tie, and underwear, which I left in a heap on the floor. He lay there naked, his skin fiery, still unable to speak.

What sort of illness took away your power of speech? Back in my childhood neighborhood, some of the fathers had suffered "nervous breakdowns" (or so they were called) when they lost their jobs or had extramarital affairs that soured. They'd disappear for days, sometimes drinking themselves into the hospital. One, I recalled, had even been rumored to cross-dress. Eventually they'd resurface, chastened and withdrawn. Could this be what was wrong with John: a classic nervous breakdown?

The new job, the new baby, money woes—clearly, it had all been too much. One night not long before, he'd arrived home from work with the back of his pants soaked, not with sweat, but with loose feces—a situation he said was due to fierce side effects caused by new medication his psychiatrist had prescribed. He'd also tripped over that weight at the gym, and the prior weekend, when Robert and Nancy had come for brunch, he'd developed a bizarre case of hiccups that shook the rafters and wouldn't quit. It was mostly funny—we'd tried every crazy trick in the book to get them to stop. He'd finally called his internist, who had diagnosed (what else?) stress and prescribed belladonna, an operatic-sounding remedy that succeeded in quickly shutting them down.

In the previous year, John had also had chicken pox, which he had caught from Caroline because apparently he'd never had it as a kid. It knocked him out for a full two weeks with a fever and zillions of angry red sores. According to the doctor, this was the typical reaction of an adult to the childhood disease. Soon after recovering, John had complained of pains "like needles" in his chest, and I'd rushed him to the emergency room at St. Vincent's Hospital, where they diagnosed pleurisy, an inflammation of the lining of the pleural cavity around the lungs. An antibiotic cleared it right up, so we didn't dwell on it.

I wasn't the only one to notice John's nagging illnesses and dark mood—my adoring parents had also sensed a crack in the firmament. A few days after Daniel was born we'd headed down to see them in Philadelphia for the weekend, and all John had wanted to do was sit on their front steps and smoke one Merit cigarette after another. "What's wrong with him?" my father had asked, gazing from his dining room window out at John's solitary figure. "Nothing, Dad!" I'd snapped. Didn't he know how hard John was working on the new *Journal* section? So much was riding on it, including his professional future, not to mention his—our—paycheck.

Now, back at our condo, John's skin was scorching to the touch. I started for a thermometer in the bathroom, but was stopped by plaintive whimpers coming from the baby monitor. I rushed to my newborn son in the front bedroom, lifted his tiny form out of the crib, unbuttoned my blouse, unfastened my damp nursing bra, and offered his tiny beak my raw, chapped nipple, feeling instantly relieved by giving him sustenance, and by his sister's even breathing in the nearby bed. If I could just stay in that Johnson & Johnson–scented sanctuary until morning, maybe this horrific night would magically disappear.

I couldn't find the thermometer, but I didn't need one; I'd never felt skin that hot. *Do nervous breakdowns cause fever?* I wondered. I considered taking John to the hospital, but what would I do with the children? As the evening raged on, I careened between believing him deathly ill and simply down with a touch of food poisoning. I picked up the phone, put it down, paced, picked it up again. I wanted to talk to someone for reassurance, but who? I'd already checked in with Robert and Nancy; beyond those trusted two, I was wary of spreading the news of John's mysterious symptoms.

Maybe it's me, I thought. I was overreacting. After all, I'd given birth just three weeks before. I retrieved our dog-eared copy of *Dr. Spock's Baby and Child Care* and found the chapter entitled "Post-partum Depression Syndrome," described as a "blue feeling" with symptoms ranging from agitation to delusion. That was me: agitated with a capital A. Thinking John was deathly ill, when all he probably had was the flu. I just needed to talk to a doctor for reassurance. I remembered John's new psychiatrist, Dr. Cooper. I raced into our back office, where I rifled through John's neat stack of bills and found a piece of letterhead from the doctor's office. I called, left a message with his service, then hung up and waited, rocking nervously in the springy Aeron chair. Within minutes, the phone rang. I lurched for it, knocking over a cold cup of coffee.

"Mrs. Andrew? This is Dr. Cooper."

"Dr. Cooper, I took John out for dinner tonight, and he, well, he couldn't talk—couldn't use the right words! He thought an ashtray was a ketchup bottle!"

The psychiatrist calmly advised me to let John sleep. Assuming he was well enough, he'd see John at their appointment the very next morning, when he could evaluate him.

I hung up, feeling a tsunami of relief. Maybe Dr. Cooper had seen this sort of thing in lots of people. Maybe an extremely virulent strain of flu was going around, setting everybody on their ears. John and I would look back on this night years from now and elbow each other, laughing, as we shared the harrowing story of his twenty-four-hour Mongolian flu.

Overcome by hope, I determined to revive him. I charged into the bedroom, tore off my clothes, and climbed onto him, shoving my tongue into his fiery mouth. "C'mon, John!" I begged. "*C'mon!*"

But he was a rag doll. Lifeless.

Hello, Baby,

I bought a chicken, which I will broil tonight. Do not worry about Bill or money or our future or anything else, please. Everything will be Tootie Wootie.

Love you, Johnski

Three

The next morning, I opened one gummy eye to see John at the mirror, showered, dressed, and methodically knotting a vibrant foulard tie as if nothing had happened. My husband had rejoined the land of the living! I sprung up to feel his cool forehead and pulled him close. "Hey!" he exclaimed, holding his tie with one hand and putting his other arm around me for ballast.

"How do you feel today?" I heard myself nearly shout.

"Okay," he replied. "I just need some coffee."

I launched into quizzing him about the night before. Did he remember not calling things by their right names?

John shrugged. "I'm just so tired."

I pressed. "I was really worried, so I called Dr. Cooper. I'm so glad you have an appointment with him this morning!" I said, masking my anxiety with pep.

"Why did you call Cooper?" he snapped, heading for the kitchen. "I'm fine."

I plopped back down on the bed. Had he no recollection

of last night? I grabbed my robe and padded into the kitchen, where John was meticulously spooning coffee into our Melitta, then bustling from the silverware drawer to the refrigerator to the cabinet for mugs. His swift actions fairly crackled with energy. I could hardly believe my eyes.

John smiled up at me. "Juice?" he asked, taking two glasses over to the table, his shiny black brogues clicking on the hardwood floor. He whipped open his morning paper, which, miraculously, he'd walked down three steep flights to retrieve.

How could John be so utterly revived? I threw my arms around his shoulders, savoring the feel of his strong muscles beneath the crisp oxford cloth.

"Hey!" he kidded, reaching around and grabbing one of my wrists. My John was here. He was back!

I poured myself some coffee and, before I could take my first gulp, spied a tousled little blonde toddling toward me, her chubby arms outstretched. "Up, Mommy! Behfast!" As if on cue, whimpers crackled on her brother's baby monitor. The normal cacophony of the day had begun.

John drained his cup, put on his suit jacket, retrieved his briefcase, and bent down to kiss me on the forehead with lips so cool they couldn't possibly have been the same scorching ones from the night before. He kissed Caroline, too, on what he liked to call her *keppie*, or *keppelah* ("head," in Yiddish), a favorite word of mine. "Bye, Daddy!" she said.

Halfway out the door, John reminded me that he was off to Dr. Cooper before work, and at noon, a birthday lunch with Robert. He'd call me sometime in between. Then, with what I swear was a spring in his step, he was off.

The apartment was still, except for Caroline slurping her Cheerios and Dan's contented suckling noises at my breast. Everything seemed astonishingly under control. I looked over at a childhood photo of John on the bookshelf and smiled. The contrast between my strong, handsome husband and that undersized, lonely-looking boy always touched me deeply. We were kindred spirits, John and me—both ugly ducklings who became swans. I had felt oversize as a child; he was undersize. When he was in junior high, fresh from a trip to the orthodontist for brand-new braces, his mother had sent him to the local store for milk, where he'd run into some popular girls from school. One had snickered, "Oh, God, glasses, red hair, pimples—and now braces, too?" In high school, some cool guys had once invited John to play a round of golf at a neighborhood course. John knew little about golf, yet had intrepidly agreed to meet them. When he got there, they were nowhere to be found. He'd been "punked."

There was never much comfort at home after such incidents, as John's uncompromising father picked up where the abusers left off. After high school, John defied Merle by attending Brown instead of Harvard, where he could finally stretch his eclectic, sardonic, style-savvy genius wings. At Brown, John—affectionately known as "Johnny A."—spent most of his time writing for and editing the school's daily newspaper. A video from his freshman year shows him clowning around the school's verdant campus, his vibrant hair cascading over his shoulders. It is one of just a handful of photos I've seen from his youth that show him smiling. At Brown, John was happy.

After graduation, he snagged a plum copywriting job at J. Walter Thompson in Chicago. A subsequent stint at Harvard

Business School confirmed that he didn't want to be in business at all, unless it was the business of newspapers, and he was promptly hired as a reporter by *The Wall Street Journal*'s Los Angeles bureau. After that, there was no stopping him. It was John's lifeblood to put the news out, put it out first, and do it well— particularly investigative stories that exposed the truth about corporate dishonesty or villainy. I loved that about him: how hard he toiled on the side of good.

Now, he was back, my John, miraculously recovered from the night before. A few hours later, I nearly skipped across Washington Street to Maxwell's for lunch with my old friend Andy, the prototypically good-looking older brother of a college roommate, in town on business.

I burst into the restaurant and Andy's broad, blazered form encased me in a bear hug. We chatted about the new baby, I showed him pictures, and when he asked after John I found myself spilling the traumatic details of not just the night before, but the stressful months leading up to it.

Andy took a long draw of Chardonnay. "Epstein-Barr," he said. "Sounds like Epstein-Barr."

Epstein-Barr was a virus everyone was abuzz about. I'd recently heard about it from my parents; a young daughter of their friend had been debilitated by it, unable to attend school for an entire year. Apparently, Andy's friend had also just been diagnosed with it; like John, she had been tired, achy, stressed, and presenting multiple symptoms, including swollen glands and rashes, for months.

Like John. Yes, just like John!

According to Andy, Epstein-Barr was manageable—even curable—with the proper treatment. His friend was nearly back to her old self. Oh, the day was going to be a good one! I let myself have not just one but two celebratory glasses of wine.

After lunch, feeling no pain, I made my way across the bustling boulevard back to the condo, where twelve-year-old Michelle, one of the girls from the condo downstairs who frequently babysat, handed me my sweaty, sleepy son. "We just got back from the park," she said. "You have a lot of messages on the machine."

A lot of messages? My euphoria evaporated as I rushed to the phone. The number 9 flashed insistently on the answering machine. My heart stopped.

Stay calm, stay calm. I fished around my pocketbook for dollars and shoved them into Michelle's hand, ushering her to the door. The bottom of my skirt was being tugged. I looked down to see Caroline's hot, red little face. "Mommy, book!"

"In a minute, honey." I shifted Dan to my other hip. Sweat pouring, hands trembling, I punched "play."

12:20 p.m: "Mrs. Andrew, this is Dr. Cooper. Can you please give me a call? The number is…"

12:30 p.m: "Maggie, this is Robert. Call me."

12:33 p.m: "Mrs. Andrew, this is Dr. Cooper again. Give me a call, please?"

1:02 pm: "Mrs. Andrew, this is admissions at Mount Sinai Hospital. Please call us at…"

1:15 p.m: *Click.*

1:25 p.m: "Mrs. Andrew, this is Dr. Rothstein at Mount Sinai Hospital. I'm calling about your husband, John Andrew. Please give me a call when you receive this message."

1:35 p.m: *Click.*

1:45 p.m: *Click.*

1:50 p.m: *Click.*

"Mommy!" Caroline glared up at me, her face stained with tears. I took her little hand and settled her in front of our small television with a bag of Doritos, then returned to the answering machine.

I dialed Dr. Cooper, who picked up immediately. In a measured tone, he explained how, when he'd met with John that morning, he'd found him to be behaving normally, though exhausted. It was only at the end, when John had written the wrong amount and date on his check in a shaky hand, that he'd grown concerned enough to arrange a brain scan for him at Mount Sinai Hospital that afternoon.

"It's just a precaution," he said. "Probably Mount Sinai has even called you by now with the results? They'll have answers. Stay in touch. We'll talk soon. Good luck."

Good luck. Good luck with what?

I punched back through the messages and dialed Dr. Rothstein at Mount Sinai Hospital.

"Dr. Rothstein's office," a female voice answered.

The inside of my mouth felt like dry paste. I wet my lips, swallowed, and managed to string together the words "This is Mrs. Andrew returning Dr. Rothstein's call."

A pause, then a booming male voice. "Mrs. Andrew, how are you?"

"Okay," I croaked.

"Mrs. Andrew," he continued, almost buoyantly, "we've performed a brain scan on your husband, John, and have detected some lesions."

Lesions? "What does that mean?"

"Well, we can't know at this point," he answered. "They could indicate something we call lymphoma, a form of cancer. We'll need to do more tests. I'm going to admit him for a few days."

Suddenly, a panorama of the past difficult year came into view. Rashes. Pleurisy. Fatigue. Swollen ankles. Explosive diarrhea. Depression. And out of my trembling lips came a voice that didn't sound like mine.

"Could he have AIDS?" I heard myself ask. The question came unpremeditated: even I was surprised by it.

A few seconds passed. "Why do you ask, Mrs. Andrew?"

"Because everything is wrong with him."

Maggie,

Dearest darling, you are a wonderful mother and sexy, loving, skinny wife. And you are still—and always—the original spark of life. I will always support you in whatever you want to do.

All my love, John

Four

W hy *had* I asked the doctor that? Not once, during any of John's illnesses, had I doubted they were anything more than what every doctor—from the internist to the gastroenterologist, the dermatologist, and the psychiatrist—had said: stress. True, he was always a little sick, but until the night before, it had never been anything eventful, just annoying, persistent little intestinal bugs and skin maladies. And yes, he was dead tired at night, but so were we both. We were overstretched, sleep-deprived young parents. When or where has there been a young parent who wasn't?

In the end, any time John had been sick in our six years together, he'd seen a doctor, and not one of those doctors had ever suggested AIDS. Why would such a thing even enter my mind? Yet, on the phone with Dr. Rothstein, each of those illnesses had flashed into one chilling snapshot: a picture of everyone I'd ever known, or heard about, dying of AIDS.

Back in the early eighties, during my dalliance with theater and waitressing, the guys in dance class had whispered about a mysterious "gay cancer." At the restaurant, one of the waiters had caught a bad cold that turned into pneumonia. He took to wearing layers of pancake makeup; rumor had it that it was to "cover up sores." He missed a day or two of work, then a stretch of them, then we didn't see him again.

"He's really sick," someone had said.

"It's AIDS," someone else said.

It wasn't long before two more waiters followed suit, suffering a string of illnesses and then disappearing entirely.

"Mrs. Andrew?" said Dr. Rothstein, "you still there?" I was, barely. He said something about running John's blood through some tests, that he'd call back when he knew something more. I stood with the receiver in one hand, a sleeping, sweaty baby— mine, apparently—slipping from the crook of my other arm.

No, the idea was ridiculous. Impossible. But if John *did* have AIDS, did the baby have it, too? I looked at Caroline, splayed on the crumby carpet transfixed by the flickering TV, her apple cheeks smeared orange with Dorito dust. Did she have it?

Did I have it?

Were we all dying?

No, I told myself. *John can't have AIDS. He isn't gay.*

When it came to AIDS in 1990 Hoboken, we were all pretty sure we knew the score. It had become a full-blown epidemic, killing thousands of gay men. Headlines had begun to report celebrities, including actor Rock Hudson and designer Perry Ellis, dying of it. Randy Shilts's book *And the Band Played On: Politics, People, and the AIDS Epidemic* was flying off the shelves, and rabble-rousing gay men's organizations such as ACT UP and the Gay Men's Health Crisis (GMHC) were gaining steam. Just a short ferry ride away, to walk down any street in Greenwich Village was to chance a skeletal young man coming at you, lurching along on his cane with haunted, sunken eyes and purple spots on his face. You'd abruptly shift your gaze and pretend to be fascinated by a shop window across the street; you didn't want to see walking death on a bright, sunny day. God help you if you were worried about getting sick like that because you were a gay man, or because your lover had suddenly become ill. God help you if your beloved family member or friend was suffering in this way. AIDS. Horrible.

But AIDS only affected gay men—the kind who wore chaps and bandannas, and had keys hanging off their belt loops, like the Village People. The kind who engaged in high-risk, unprotected sex in back-street downtown clubs. Right?

Of course, we also knew people who'd died of AIDS who didn't look at all like that—coworkers, cousins, uncles, brothers—some who'd "come out," others who hadn't but were considered terminally single, asexual, or "light." After a few beers, the men in our crowd referred to these men as "three-dollar bills" and "taking it up the keister for Easter." In reference to a popular Manhattan health club, they joked, "Don't pick up the soap!" And we'd all read sad accounts about gay men infected by the disease who'd been shunned by family and friends, fired from jobs, and, in some cases, beaten senseless.

We still weren't exactly sure how you contracted AIDS—many were afraid to kiss gay friends or use their bathrooms. But we didn't think about it all that much. We were married, our Hoboken crowd, and—it went without saying at that time—straight. AIDS was the last thing we had to worry about. Except, in the Y locker room the other day, hadn't my friend Linda mentioned a story she'd seen on the news about a woman catching AIDS from her dentist? And what about that girl, Ali Gertz, whom we'd read about in *The New York Times*? Twenty-three, white, upper-middle-class, Jewish, and educated at Horace Mann, this girl had contracted AIDS from a date with a heterosexual guy seven years before. What if you'd slept with someone a long time ago who unknowingly carried the AIDS virus and he gave it to you—how would you even know you had it? There was also the *Starsky and Hutch* actor Paul Michael Glaser's wife, Elizabeth, who'd contracted AIDS from a blood transfusion and passed it on to her daughter through breastfeeding. Their little girl had died of AIDS two years before.

But none of this had anything to do with John. He wasn't gay. He'd had a long-term girlfriend before me, after all. He was also, hands down, the best lover I'd ever had. It didn't matter where or when: John was tear-your-clothes-off desirous. I thought back to the first time we'd had sex after Caroline's birth. After six weeks of abstinence prescribed by the doctors, I'd called John to tell him I had the all-clear. Within what seemed like minutes he'd burst into the apartment, torn off his clothes, and pushed me down onto the hardwood floor. His lust and love had cascaded over me, the room musty with the scent of our heat. Afterward he'd managed to return to work, but that evening found him hobbling to the corner pharmacy for Doan's Pills: oh, his aching back. We laughed so hard—and then fell into bed again, and again. This was how John was with sex—never able to wait, never getting enough. Gay men didn't sleep with women as hungrily, as lustfully, as John did with me. Did they?

On the other hand, John wasn't exactly a conventional guy—a "guy's guy." He never spent Sunday on the couch glued to a bowl game on TV, or tossing a Frisbee around the park. He read books, steamed lobsters, drank wine, and happily tagged along with me to dance concerts. And there was that body of his. As a failed dancer who could never be thin enough, I was in awe of John's impeccable build and the amount of sweat he put into keeping it that way: regular trips to the gym and intricate work-outs based on muscle-magazine spreads. His disciplined attention to the attainment of an aesthetic ideal was something I'd seen in few men other than many of the dancers and actors I'd known. They all possessed an undeniable "cock of the walk" confidence and allure, not to mention the washboard abs and tight butts that I saw in John. They were all gay.

And there was John's pile of muscle magazines—they stuck in my craw. How many ways were there to tone a tricep? The look of the men modeling in these magazines: they weren't cool or "camp" like everything else in John's life. They were badly photographed, overly lubed cartoon superheroes wearing cheesy leopard-print bikini briefs. People like these crass Mr. Universes would normally cause John to roll his eyes and smirk. So why couldn't he get enough of them? It was something I didn't want to think about, him poring over those magazines.

One day early in our relationship, lying beside John in post-coital reverie, I had felt the need to ask him if he'd ever slept with men. It wasn't AIDS I was worried about back in 1984. But I wanted to know—needed to know. Back then, you were either straight, gay, or bi. Not that you'd admit to the last two.

"No," John had answered, without missing a beat.

I'd nuzzled his neck, relieved, and enthusiastically climbed on top of him. Suddenly he'd pushed me away and looked me in the eyes. "You? Women?"

"No," I'd replied. "I mean, there was this one time in summer stock when I was asked, but, you know, I said no because I had no interest in sex with women. I only cared about having sex with…you," I said, burrowing into his pulsating flesh. "It's *you* I want, it's you I…" I trailed off, unable to speak as he traced an imaginary line from my breastbone, down, down, down.

John. The best lover, ever. All mine.

Of course, the past few months hadn't been exactly Club Hedonism. We'd each been into our own things, John working like a dog every day on the new section and me hauling my pregnant carcass around the stage of a local church every night, choreographing a musical: two ships passing in the night. Who had the time, or energy, for sex?

No, John wasn't gay. He also hadn't had a blood transfusion, nor was he an intravenous drug user: the other people out there getting AIDS. People like that hung around back alleys and kept strange hours, didn't they? John was home every night like clockwork and rarely left the office during the workday. I knew, because I called incessantly, asking what he wanted for dinner or to share something cute about Caroline. If he was out, he was at a business meeting, the gym, or a private class. John was a lesson junkie. In the six years since we'd met, he'd not only written and published a book—on municipal bonds, dedicated to me!—but had taken up windsurfing and jazz piano, sewn a pair of pants, taught himself to install track lighting, and after a number of dogged attempts, managed to achieve perfect pesto.

Perfect pesto, perfect body. Or rather, bodies. Perfect bodies. I thought back to a moment I'd tried to forget.

About a month before Dan was born, John took Caroline and me for a swim at his pool. His latest self-improvement project was to become a better swimmer, and he'd begun doing laps every day at the Battery Park Swim and Health Club near his office. He'd even retained a lifeguard on staff named Jose to help him fine-tune his kicks and strokes.

It was a steamy Saturday in May. At eight months pregnant, I was big as a proverbial house. Stretched across my swollen protuberance was the ugliest piece of rayon ever designed, a borrowed maternity bathing suit that wouldn't even make a gestating Christie Brinkley look good.

We arrived at the pool and had barely flip-flopped our way onto its deck when John called out to an impressively bronzed and ripped figure atop the lifeguard stand: "Jose! Hi!" It was more unbridled enthusiasm than I'd seen in John for...how long?

"Hey, John!" The muscular form waved back, swinging himself over his seat and scampering down the ladder. Sleek and sinewy, Jose approached the three of us smiling.

"How you doin', man?" he asked, clasping John's hand—or was it his forearm, or were they now hugging? Yes. It was that sort of half–arm wrestle, half-hug thing that men...some men...did.

After a second or two, John broke away and said, "I want you to meet my wife and daughter."

I could feel Caroline's shy face pressed against the backs of my sweaty, meaty knees, and wished I could hide there, too. Jose extended his callused hand. "Hello, Mrs. Andrew," he said.

I always hated being called that. It wasn't my name. Not his fault, but still. And I hated how alike and symbiotic he and John looked, standing there side by side, their chiseled physiques complemented by tiny Speedos. I always thought John wore a Speedo to swim faster. Aerodynamics, I think it was called.

But I also had another thought, by no means a comfortable one. I'd realized, suddenly, that I was the odd man out.

Oh, God.

I had filed that forlorn pool scene, which had been quite painful at the time, away in an imaginary folder labeled, "It's nothing. Don't worry about it." Labeled, I now slowly realized, "Denial."

"Moooommmmyyy!" my daughter yelled from her position in front of the TV. "I'm *hungwy*, I said!"

What time was it? I looked down at my watch. Five o'clock! It had been more than an hour since my phone conversation with the doctor. I shook myself.

"Mommy!" Caroline was now at my feet, her mouth quivering.

"Caroline, honey, I'm sorry," I said, picking up her sturdy little form. "Mommy had to talk on the phone. I'll make you hot dogs and macaroni, okay?"

"When Daddy home?" she asked.

Caroline loved her daddy. Every night he read to her from their favorite book, *One Fish, Two Fish, Red Fish, Blue Fish*, delighting in the line "And lots of good fun that is funny." He'd recently taken Caroline to his office to show her off, where they'd giggled over a Xerox of the fluffy behind of Caroline's beloved stuffed dog, Charlotte. It was, of course, John, with his droll sense of humor, who'd given that dirty, floppy dog such an uncannily proper name. A couple years earlier, John had taken Caroline and Charlotte to pick up groceries at a gourmet food shop a few towns over, returning hours later with the food and Caroline—but no Charlotte. You never saw anybody move faster than John that day, racing down the winding flights of the condo, charging out to his Datsun, and zooming off to rescue his daughter's beloved toy.

"Daddy's not coming home tonight," I said.

"Why?"

"He had to go on a trip." The lies were off and running.

"Why?"

I surrendered to an endless round of "Why?" and "Because" while I fed and bathed her, then plunked her down again in front of the ever-loving television.

AIDS. A wave of panic came over me.

In the fading light of evening, my image of the disease came sharply into focus. Though I suffered the same misconceptions as everyone, I had seen its effects firsthand among my singing waiter group. The most gifted of them, my dear friend Chris, had died of AIDS-related illnesses only the previous spring.

Chris and his boyfriend, Steve, had lived on a charming little stretch of West 13th Street in the Village. Chris and I sang and waited tables together, wearing marinara-stained aprons printed with "Make a cow happy, eat fish today!" After our shifts, we'd close down the place, drinking cheap wine and smoking pot. When I was eventually cast in a regional dinner theater production and Chris was cast as the lead in a national tour of *Joseph and the Amazing Technicolor Dreamcoat*, we saw less of each other. I did summer stock, met John, and got married; Chris continued his life on the road. Once in a while, I'd get a letter. "Miss you," he'd write.

One chilly April day in 1988, just after Caroline was born, Chris came by to meet her. His normally glowing face was ghostly and he stifled a cough.

"It's just a cold," Chris protested when I expressed concern. He was full of his usual energy and his warm brown eyes shone, especially while he was holding my child. What a sweetheart he was.

Soon afterward, Chris landed an overseas tour of *South Pacific* while I became consumed with mothering and domesticity. We lost touch.

Two years later, pregnant again, I was reclining on the living room couch, my swollen feet propped up on the coffee table, when the phone rang. It was Steve. "Chris is in the hospital," he said, "and he doesn't have long." It was AIDS.

I dialed John at work, my heart racing. "Chris is dying of AIDS at St. Vincent's," I said. "I've got to go."

The next day, John and I drove to the hospital. After several minutes looking for a parking spot, he swerved into an illegal space across from the hospital and lit up a Merit. As usual, John would never pay for parking. A bespoke suit for himself, or an occasional lavish gift for me? Sure. But a parking garage? Never.

"You know, baby," he said, "it's been a long week. Why don't I sit here and stay with the car while you go see Chris? He probably just wants to see you, anyway."

I looked at him, taking a drag of his cigarette. What was up here? Was he afraid of being close to someone with AIDS? A lot of people were. I was the pregnant one, though—shouldn't I have been afraid? But then, we both knew the virus didn't fly through the air. I steeled myself, popped open the car door, lifted my heft up and out of the low-slung Datsun, and crossed the street to the hospital.

In the room that was supposed to be Chris's, there was a shriveled old man shivering in one of the beds. "Chris?" I ventured. He slowly turned his head and focused his alert, beautiful brown eyes on mine.

"Chris," I said.

"Hi, sweetie," he croaked.

I hugged his sack of bones and sat with him, holding a cup to his cracked lips. His face was burning hot but his stiff little hands were ice cold. I'd never seen anyone that ill.

After a few minutes, I ran out of things to tell him about my absurdly carefree existence. I was swollen with life, while he, at just twenty-seven, was at the end of his. I stood up to leave and leaned over to kiss his lined, sweaty forehead. "I love you," I said.

"I love you, too," he whispered, closing his eyes.

Big as I was, I bolted for the elevator and nearly broke the down button, pounding on it until the doors opened to take me to the lobby. I rammed every pound of my swollen might against the revolving door and burst out into the fresh spring air, gasping. John was there, waiting in the car where I'd left him.

"How was he?" he asked.

"Awful! He—it—was awful," I reported, shaking, unable to make sense of the ghoulish transformation of my once vibrant, magnificent friend.

John put his cigarette in his mouth and placed his strong yet soft hand on mine. "Let's go out for dinner," he suggested. He revved the motor and zoomed us to a nearby bistro he liked, where, as luck would have it, a parking spot opened up just as we arrived.

I was seven months pregnant, but nothing could keep me from knocking back two glasses of Pinot Grigio that night, surgeon general's warnings be damned. I remember clasping John's hand across the table and feeling safe, warm, and loved in that softly lit restaurant, so close to and yet so far from the St. Vincent's Hospital AIDS ward. And feeling lucky. So lucky.

The phone rang.

"Mrs. Andrew? Dr. Rothstein. We don't know anything definitive yet," he said. "But we do want you in for an AIDS test. Tomorrow morning, ten-thirty." He recited the office address. "Okay? Then, I'd like to see you here at the hospital sometime tomorrow afternoon."

The room swayed. They wanted me to take an AIDS test? I grabbed the edge of the table to keep from falling. "Nope," I barked hoarsely, then cleared my throat. "No. Did you know I just had a baby? I have another child, too, a little girl. She has a swimming lesson tomorrow morning, and I have to take her. So, no, I can't do it—can't go tomorrow at ten-thirty. Also, I live in Hoboken. So—no. Can't do it."

"Mrs. Andrew, I'm very sorry about this, really I am. But you need to show up at that office tomorrow morning. We strongly urge you to get there," he said. "Please."

"Okay," I said. I hung up and walked to the front room to check on the baby, who was sleeping soundly. I returned to the TV room, scooped the peacefully snoring Caroline off the floor, and carried her back to the tiny front room to tuck her into her bed beside Dan's crib. I put my hand on my son's moist back and felt the purr of his contented breath.

My babies.

"Please, God, don't let them be sick," I prayed. I went to the phone and called my parents.

I love you, baby, and let's go skiing sometime.
John

Five

Hearing my father's familiar gravelly voice made me weak with relief.

"Kila!" he called, covering the phone. My father often called my mother, Carolyn, by her Yiddish name. She'd be downstairs washing or ironing, and despite her seventy-two years, I knew once she was aware it was me calling, she'd trip up the basement's linoleum steps to their living room phone in hopes of being regaled with a cute anecdote about her grandchildren. In these days before smartphones, FaceTime, and texting, such calls were worth their weight in gold.

"Hi, Mag!" she sang. My mother's voice had a perpetual lilt. The earth could be swallowing her whole and she'd still be smiling beatifically. She never let sadness show; there was always a steely resolve, a best foot forward.

How do you tell your parents that your husband, your classy Ivy League trophy, the father of their grandchildren, a young man primed to become managing editor of one of the country's major newspapers, a man more son than son-in-law, might have AIDS?

"John is sick," I said.

"Oh?" asked my father.

I choked out the details of the birthday dinner disaster and all that had spiraled down since, including John's potential diagnosis. They were quiet for a moment. "Oh," my father said.

"Hold on, Mag," he continued. "Kila!" he shouted, forgetting my mother was on the line. "We have to pack!"

"Dad," I cried out, nausea surging up, "what am I going to do if it *is* AIDS? What if we're all sick?"

"Just hold on, Mag," he said. He told me they'd get there as soon possible, and rushed off the phone.

From then on, my parents became my angels. I was in trouble and needed them desperately. Trouble they knew; trouble they could handle. Their generation had seen it all. What was so bad compared to two world wars, the Great Depression, the Holocaust, the loss of so many they'd loved? I didn't realize what a uniquely useful quality this was, the unwavering resilience of my parents, until John's illness.

The next morning I got up and, in preparation for my AIDS test, was surprised to feel the need to clean up. I certainly couldn't wear my uniform of the past post-partum weeks: stretched-out, oversize tees stained with formula and spit-up. In the back of my closet I came across an elegant black Henri Bendel ensemble that I'd forgotten I owned; a splurge for a memorable date with John soon after we were married. It had been a party, hosted by a co-worker who'd rented his downtown loft to Paramount Pictures for their 1987 hit movie *Fatal Attraction*. The loft was in Manhattan's Meatpacking District, a neighborhood not yet dominated by the Standard Hotel and Kardashian look-alikes (if not the real thing) but by slaughterhouses, seedy bars, gay clubs, and prostitutes. At the party were John's horn-rimmed colleagues mixed with electric people from the neighborhood: drag queens, models, and celebrities. We danced as though possessed to David Byrne wailing "Psycho Killer." Afterward, desperate for scrambled eggs, we staggered across Gansevoort Street to Florent, a legendary twenty-four-hour bistro whose proprietor, Florent Morellet, had AIDS and famously posted his T-cell count (the white cells that help fight off disease) on the menu board above his blue-plate special. AIDS had seemed so alien that night. Them, not us.

Now, once again clad in my chic Bendel ensemble, I found myself sitting in a Park Avenue doctor's waiting room surrounded by skinny young men. One had an eye patch; another was hooked up to an IV. None of us spoke or looked at one another. Toes were tapping, legs twitching, magazine pages being thumbed. Attendants dozed.

I was ushered into an examining room where a nurse, her eyes full of pity, asked me to step on the scale. I'd lost six pounds in the past week. When, again, was the last time I ate?

She directed me to roll up one sleeve of my blouse and began preparing the syringe to draw blood when three young, lab-coated interns slipped into the room. Here was an interesting, unusual case to observe, they must have thought: a woman, and a mother. You didn't hear about too many women getting AIDS, other than a few celebrities, the woman infected by her dentist, and that girl who caught it from her bad date.

A man who appeared to be close to my age, despite an avuncular-looking mustache, entered the examining room. Though not wearing a doctor's traditional white coat, he introduced himself as Dr. Eric Neibart. He briskly donned latex gloves and asked me to make a fist. He took the syringe from the nurse and inserted it into my vein.

"We won't know your results until tomorrow afternoon," he said. "Come see me in my office before you leave." He patted my shoulder and left.

Doctors had been patting me a lot lately.

The interns filed out behind him. They were probably fresh from Harvard and Hopkins; confident, smug, the world at their feet. I wanted to shout at them: *My husband works at* The Wall Street Journal! *He went to a great college, just like you. So did I! We have a daughter and, three weeks ago, I just had another baby. Everyone sent me flowers and gifts! I grew up in the suburbs and have a normal life. I am not supposed to be here. Don't you for one minute think I am!*

Afterward, a nurse ushered me into Dr. Neibart's office, where he sat behind a large, immaculate desk. We dispensed with the formalities.

"Mrs. Andrew," he said, "John's test results are not yet conclusive, but we have good reason to believe he has AIDS."

My nausea switched back on. It was becoming like breathing.

"Do you think I have it, too?" I asked weakly. "And what about the kids?"

Dr. Neibart asked when my son had been born and his weight. I told him as he scribbled on his clipboard. "A baby that big could be an indicator of your own good health," he said. "And when did you last have sex with your husband?"

I knew the answer: it had been four months ago, on a business trip in Florida. We'd laughed uproariously that night about my huge pregnant belly; was it a fullback in there? John would need a crane to do it! I also remembered we'd used a condom, as John had had an outbreak of herpes. This bit of information caused Dr. Neibart to jot more notes on his chart, his chiseled jaw relaxing slightly when I said "condom."

In the early eighties, we had all worried about genital herpes. Nagging, communicable, and recurring, it came close to being a deal breaker in many relationships, including ours. One night, about two weeks after we'd met, and after several nights of pretty fabulous sex, John had hesitated before falling into bed.

"I have something to tell you," he'd said, taking out a condom. "I have herpes." Until then, we'd used only my diaphragm for contraception.

He explained that he'd had an outbreak that day and could protect me with the condom, adding that he was always aware when it erupted and would be vigilant about keeping me safe.

I freaked out and, for the first time in our blossoming relationship, demurred about having sex.

"What am I now, damaged goods?" he'd responded. "It's pretty uncool of you to react that way."

I'd abruptly left, spending a confused twenty-four hours mulling over my rotten luck: an amazing new boyfriend—with herpes. The problem was, I loved having sex with John, and was beginning to love him. He was right: who was I to consider him "damaged goods"? Any one of us out there having sex could have contracted it.

I called him the next day. He told me he'd caught herpes from an old girlfriend, that he had it well under control, and that if we used condoms when it erupted—which was, he said, "not that often"—I'd be fine. That night, we slept together, using a condom. I soon got over it. We used condoms a lot.

"The fact that you used condoms a lot is *very* good news," Dr. Neibart said. "What kind of condoms, do you know?" he asked, explaining that only latex, not lambskin, was effective in preventing HIV transmission.

My pulse picked up. *There were different kinds of condoms?* What kind *did* we use? I hadn't a clue.

Dr. Neibart told me to meet him the next day at two-thirty sharp for the results of my test, which he would deliver in person. If I tested HIV-negative, he explained, my children would be negative, too, as the virus was passed on to babies by their mothers during pregnancy, birth, or breastfeeding. Babies didn't get AIDS from their fathers. Or at least, not directly from their fathers.

Dr. Neibart paused. "How would your husband have gotten AIDS, Mrs. Andrew? Do you know?"

I shook my head. Again, I hadn't a clue.

Before dismissing me, Dr. Neibart asked if I had a psychiatrist. He scribbled something on another pad, tore it off, and gave it to me. "Call her," he said. "She's good."

Welcome to the wonderful world of AIDS, I thought. A world I never imagined would be mine.

When I got home, I paid the babysitter and settled back on the couch to nurse Dan, pushing away my worry about passing HIV on to him. I would feed my hungry son, I *would*. Little Caroline perched next to me, sucking a lollipop. She had her priorities straight. I had begun to unfasten my nursing bra when a flashing light caught my eye: the answering machine. Once again, there were nine messages. I stabbed its playback button.

8:00 a.m: "Hi, Mag. Where were you yesterday? I'm leaving for the Y and am not running without you today. Be there!"

8:10 a.m: *Click.*

8:20 a.m: "Mag. Lucia. Meet me at the corner for the Y? Let me know. Bye!"

10:16 a.m: "Okay, we ran. Where were you?"

10:45 a.m. "Hi, Maggie. Michael wants to know if he can play with Caroline today?"

And so on. I couldn't call any of my friends back. What would I say? "Hi, John's in the hospital. He has AIDS. See you soon!"

Dr. Rothstein had also called, reminding me to meet him at the hospital that day. "Four o'clock okay?"

I would have to go. John was there. It was high time I faced him.

The buzzer sounded. My parents! I was never so happy to see them. Caroline scampered over and threw her little arms around my father's dependable, sturdy legs. While I fed them cheese sandwiches and coffee, we shared our incredulity as to how any of this could be happening. My mother set down her cup. "There's actually something John recently told me that I should share with you," she said. A few days after Dan was born, she recounted, she and my father had begun chatting with John about his experience in Vienna, where he'd spent his senior year of high school living at a boardinghouse. "I asked how he had liked it there," she said, "and he had responded something like this: 'I was very lonely and had no friends. There was a man upstairs who kept bothering me—kept asking me to come up.'"

"I had a funny feeling when he said that," she said. We sat in silence, unspoken questions hanging in the air.

After lunch, my dad drove me to the hospital to see Dr. Rothstein and John. As I was his only food source, the baby came, too. I clung to my sweet-smelling son for dear life; to hell with the car seat.

In the middle of the Lincoln Tunnel, I panicked anew. "What if we all have AIDS, Dad? What will I do?"

Keeping his eyes on the road, my father said, "If you all have AIDS, I'll take care of you."

To my dying day, I will never forget he said that.

At the hospital, we stepped off the elevator and almost collided with a bespectacled, balding man in a white coat. "Hello, I'm Dr. Rothstein," he said, extending his hand. "You're Mrs. Andrew? I'd like to speak with you in my office." He turned to my father. "Hello, sir. Could you please wait out here for a few minutes?"

I handed Dan over to his grandfather and followed the doctor to his office.

Dr. Rothstein looked like he'd rather have been almost anywhere else.

"I'm sorry, Mrs. Andrew, but it's confirmed," he said. "Your husband does have AIDS."

The air was still. There it was: the truth.

He went on to tell me that John didn't just have AIDS, he had what was called "full-blown AIDS." He was riddled with something called "opportunistic infection" and likely had about two weeks to live.

Two weeks to live? The night before, I had poured myself a big glass of scotch and forced myself to consider what would happen if John actually did, preposterously, have AIDS. He would be sick, I'd decided; the kids and I wouldn't. He'd soon get better and go back to work. We'd get divorced and raise our kids separately but amicably. I'd get married again and maybe have more kids. John would come for Thanksgiving. And so on. At no point in this fantasy would John die.

Dr. Rothstein then said, "Mrs. Andrew, we think Mr. Andrew has carried the HIV virus for a very long time. Seven, eight years, at least." I could tell he believed he was relaying a bit of good news: if John had contracted AIDS that long ago, there was a chance he'd been faithful to me. But at that moment, I didn't care if John had contracted the disease seven years ago, six months ago, or last week. I had to see him. I had to kill him.

Dr. Rothstein led me down the hall to John's room, where we passed my dozing father and baby son, born just three weeks before in the very same hospital. In room 612 I found John reclining in his bed, his beautiful, thick red hair splayed out on the white pillow, framing his face like fire.

I walked over to him. He didn't turn to greet me.

"John," I said, my voice hard, devoid of emotion. "You have AIDS."

No response.

"John," I repeated. "You have AIDS. How did you get it?"

John turned and stared at me with his cornflower blue eyes, once wry and cynical and smart and sexy, but now vapid. What he said next was so shocking and surreal that, to this day, I am chilled by it. He asked if I'd ever slept with Chris, who'd died at St. Vincent's Hospital the week after I'd visited.

In the nearly six years we'd been together, four of them married, I hadn't slept with anyone but John. It hadn't occurred to me to sleep with anyone but John. He was my everything.

"No, John. I did not sleep with Chris." I began to feel my back straighten and my shoulders lower. This was not the John I'd married, I realized, and I was no longer his "Magski." This was a different John. I was a different Maggie.

"How did you get AIDS, John?" I asked my husband again.

I'm not sure how long it was before he turned sharply away and said, "I slept with men in L.A."

At that, I turned on my heel and left his hospital room. I woke my father, grabbed hold of my baby, and marched us all to the elevator and out to the parking lot.

My father drove in silence. It was one of the few times in my life I saw him, an inveterate talker, a sales guy never lacking a pitch, speechless. The baby, smushed against my swollen bosom I was holding him so tight, woke up and began beating his head against me. Relentless, this kid. I unstrapped and nursed, amazed I could produce milk. Had I drunk anything besides morning coffee? Had I eaten anything? My mouth felt like cotton.

While Dan nursed, I cursed. How blind had I been, how duped? Here was a man good to my parents, kind to my brother, there when I needed him. I admired, no, make that worshipped— yes, *worshipped*—his competence in all things. No, make that genius—not competence, *genius*. I'd worshipped his genius. He was my best friend. He was the father of my children. I was sickened by his accusation. Did he even love me? Had our perfect *Thirtysomething* marriage been one horrible sham? Was I John's— what were they called, the wives gay men used as decoys—*beard*?

John had once told me he'd loved living in Los Angeles because it was so "guiltless." I'd heard him when he'd said it—I *had*. I saw Los Angeles that way, too. He'd introduced it to me on our honeymoon. Venice, with its glistening beachside muscle men. West Hollywood's pretty boys in tight pants. Beautiful people everywhere, strutting proud. L.A. Goddamn guiltless L.A. I had read somewhere that in the early 1980s, Los Angeles had been a hotbed of gay clubs—and sex—until AIDS slammed in, decimating the scene. Had John limited his experiments to those heady pre-AIDS days, only now realizing the risk? Or had he known all along—even during our honeymoon? How much had he been hiding from me, and for how long?

Back home, I told my mother about John's accusation, then stashed it away for almost twenty years. Like John's illness, it became a secret no one could know. And something I tried very hard to forget.

After I calmed down, she told me she'd taken some phone messages, including one from Norm Pearlstine, *The Wall Street Journal*'s managing editor. Why would the paper's managing editor call? John had only been out of the office for two days, and he didn't report to Norm anyway. Had word of his disease already gotten out? Maybe someone in the newsroom had heard, "Andrew is in the hospital." Then someone else, a few cubicles down, had added, "He hasn't been looking good lately. What's with those rashes?" If you want to keep something secret, keep it out of a newsroom.

It was getting dark. I put on the lights and lowered the shades.

My mother fed and bathed the children while my father, after stripping down to his yellowing T-shirt and baggy blue boxer shorts, poured us stiff scotches and began rifling through the filing cabinet in search of John's financial information. Did I know where this and that account was? he asked.

I didn't. Talk about oblivious. Talk about denial. Earth to Maggie. John handled everything—all the bills, holdings, and investments. In fact, I'd only recently learned of valuable land he'd inherited—or rather, *we'd* inherited.

About a year earlier, John had mentioned that he'd be heading up to New Hampshire with his brother, as they'd hired a surveyor to assess "the property."

"What property?" I'd asked.

He told me that when his maternal grandmother had died a decade before, he and his brother had each inherited acreage in Meredith, New Hampshire, on the banks, no less, of majestic Lake Winnipesaukee. He told me he was considering selling his half, hence the surveyor.

His half. *Our* half?

It hadn't bothered me at the time, head-over-heels in love as I was. Now I pondered *why* it hadn't bothered me. What other secrets had John kept?

There had also been his mother's Alzheimer's. Alice Hale Andrew, a demure, diminutive Smith College alumna, class of '33, who'd given to birth to John in her forties, was clearly in the throes of dementia when, six months into our courtship, I met her and his father for lunch in Manhattan. It was only as we walked to meet them at the restaurant that John had casually revealed his mother's condition.

Why had he waited so long to tell me? Some people, I'd concluded, were just inordinately private. Now I saw it as yet another piece of the pattern. Why keep that a secret? Why keep anything a secret?

"Mag! Come over here!" I snapped out of my thoughts. My

father wanted to show me something: some valuable stock options John owned. He'd also found a small life insurance policy, as well as papers indicating that John had life insurance through the *Journal*. With this and the yet unsold property in New Hampshire, for a while, at least, the kids and I would be okay. Of course, I'd have to go back to work. Would I be well enough to work, though, if I had AIDS? If. I'd soon know.

The phone rang; I jumped for it.

"Mrs. Andrew? It's Dr. Rothstein."

I checked my watch: 9:46 p.m. Why was he calling me now?

"Mrs. Andrew," he said, "I just wanted to tell you that I think you're going to be all right tomorrow. I'm not sure, but I think so. You just had a very big baby, and Dr. Neibart told me a good portion of the sex you had recently was protected. We don't have the results of the test yet, but let's just say I'm hopeful."

I thanked him profusely, hung up, and told my parents what he'd said. They encircled me in their arms, Caroline trotting over and reattaching herself to my father's legs. We all stood there huddled together in the center of the living room for several minutes, cautiously buoyed by the doctor's call.

The next day at two-thirty sharp I went to meet Dr. Neibart in a regal iron skyscraper, adjacent to the hospital, for my results. My parents and Dan were with me, while Caroline, now incessantly inquiring as to the whereabouts of Daddy, stayed home with the downstairs neighbors. Robert was there, too, with John's father, Merle, summoned from Bethesda, Maryland.

We assembled in the hospital's lounge on the appointed floor. When I spotted Dr. Neibart stepping off the elevator down the hall, I ran to him. He ran to me, too, sweeping me up and announcing, "You're negative! You and the children are fine!"

I collapsed into his arms, thanking him repeatedly—as if he had anything to do with it—and nearly sprinted back to the group with the news. My father was ecstatic; my mother, perched straight-backed on her chair, said dramatically, "I knew you wouldn't be sick. I just knew it." Robert's worried countenance broke open with relief. Merle stood apart, looking quizzical.

"We'll need to talk more," said Dr. Neibart. "They'll be releasing John from the hospital tomorrow."

John was coming home tomorrow? With me? I began to feel panic anew but willed myself not to let it ruin my elation about the results. Everyone was to have a life. Everyone, that was, but John.

We were strange bedfellows, amassed there at Mount Sinai hospital, linked by a man in the bed down the hall: our husband, father, brother, son, and son-in-law, dying of AIDS. Not that the name of the disease would ever again be part of the conversation. Once the relief about my test subsided, first my father, then Robert took me aside to counsel me not to tell anyone about John having AIDS.

Too much was happening, too many emotions swirled around inside, for me to make sense of much. But this much was clear: no one could know.

Maggie Poo,

You looked really pretty this morning, smelling of the shower. I really do think you're beautiful even if I told Tim you were funny first. You are funny. How did the culottes go today? Your mother is a member of the "sans culottes," the French Revolutionaries who campaigned on a platform of not wearing culottes. So here I am thinking of you. I should be writing my book, but I'd rather think of you. What can I do to help you with your transition, which will be transcendent? You have a lot of guts, and you're strong, and you have great taste in shoes.

You are sweet and sexy.

Johnski

Six

The next morning the hospital turned John over to me, along with a Hefty bag stuffed with his suit and shoes, and a Baggie containing his wallet and wedding ring. We'd dressed him in loose khakis, big enough for the diaper he had to wear, and in tennis shoes that barely fit over his swollen feet. Once we reached Hoboken, I dragged John and the bags up the steep, winding flights to our condo, where my waiting parents greeted us. Their eyes were filled with fear and as much false pep as they could muster. My dad helped me steer John into our back bedroom, and I managed to undress and scoop his hot, limp body into bed. On this sweltering summer day he was shivering, so I swathed him in a blanket and down quilt pulled from the top of the closet.

A few minutes later, out of the depths of those covers emerged the first words I had heard John utter since his terse, reluctant confession the day before.

"Now everyone will know Andrew has AIDS," he said, referring to himself by last name, as his colleagues did at the *Journal*. Newsroom jargon.

"Why do you say that, John?"

"Because you're going to tell them," he said.

My husband—a man who'd dedicated his life to exposing the truth—had a disease he had contracted through covert behavior he'd lied about until he couldn't lie anymore, a disease that would soon kill him and could have killed us. And his first concern was—did I get this right?—his professional reputation. Somehow I'd expected him to tell me how profoundly sorry he was. He didn't. He never would.

It's appalling how naïve I was, not just about the man I married but about the state of his illness. He'd looked dazed but fine at the hospital. Once at home, though, his killer infections took over. His brain was addled by lesions and plaque, brought on by toxoplasmosis, a disease caused by a parasite that preyed on compromised immune systems, and he reacted to everything I said as though enveloped in a fog. Due to vascular infection in his legs, he limped on swollen ankles (not from a gym accident, as he'd said). A thick white paste called thrush coated his tongue, and even his hair was gunked up with something. Yet even with all that was wrong with him, John had many more than two weeks to live. His health stabilized periodically and in fact, there were nearly nine challenging months to come.

The day after John returned home, I bathed Dan in his blue plastic tub in the sink, and then led John over, attempting to shampoo the green, sticky stuff off his scalp. Whatever it was, it wasn't budging. Thinking our local hair salon would be more successful, I put a clean shirt on John and limped all four of us over to its cute little storefront. The bell tinkled as we entered. "Hi, Gina!" I called to the sloe-eyed stylist, who regularly trimmed Caroline's blond wisps and liberally dispensed lollipops.

Gina looked at John and recoiled with horror. "We can't deal with that here," she said, darting to the back of the salon and behind a curtain. The other stylists stood staring, scissors in hand. I looked at my husband—his scalp a sticky mess, his green pallor, his unsteady gait. What had I been thinking? Red-faced, I rushed us out and nearly dragged John home and dropped him on the couch. My knees buckled and I collapsed into a kitchen chair, despondent. The sheer magnitude of our problem loomed. It was true: no one could know. No one. I was in this alone.

All that day and the next, I kept everyone inside, including my parents. I didn't take out the garbage or even move the car; screw the parking tickets. Finally, I had no choice but to venture out: the *Journal*'s Norm Pearlstine had requested I meet with him. My parents agreed to watch John and both kids. I put on my trusty Bendel outfit and scanned the apartment. Everyone seemed to be holding steady: John was in the back office in his pajamas, comatose on the floral fold-out couch. My father reclined on the living room couch, Dan curled up on his chest. And my mother, her salt-and-pepper bob caught up in a girlish ponytail, was stirring mac and cheese for Caroline, who was intently introducing fluffy Charlotte to Prom Queen Barbie.

I teetered down the three flights, my swollen post-pregnancy feet crammed into strappy sandals with pointy heels. As I pushed open the brownstone's solid oak front door, a blast of sun and heat and people assaulted me. I recoiled into the dark foyer, rummaging blindly for my sunglasses, then made a break for the bus. As we bounced down Washington Street, my engorged breasts ached. I was due to feed Dan soon. I had no makeup on, and none with me. Was my hair clean, let alone combed?

Once at the *Journal*, I headed straight for the ladies' room. I look like hell, I thought. I loaded my nursing bra with Kleenex to catch any leaks and took the high-speed elevator up to Norm's sunken living room of an office, overlooking majestic New York harbor.

Norm's secretary offered me tea. He and I sat facing each other in plush leather Knoll lounge chairs. "What's wrong with John?" he asked.

"John's very sick," I said. "He won't survive. I can't really talk about it."

I could tell that Norm didn't need any more information. He knew.

"How can I help?" he asked.

I looked at him blankly. I hadn't thought that far.

"What's happening?" he asked.

In a rush, I told him about the mounting hospital bills, the daunting task of applying for insurance reimbursement, the many appointments I had to get John to while juggling the kids. Norm picked up the phone and asked the human resources department to call him about John's insurance, then handed me an account number for the *Journal*'s car service, insisting I use it "anywhere, anytime." He also gave me a card with his home number.

I returned home in a partial reverie. Here was help. Here was no judgment, no stigma or fear. Here was a friend.

For the rest of July we limped along, our lives a macabre dance in which I bathed, fed, and diapered two babies and their father. Every day, I took John into Manhattan for appointments with his dermatologist, vascular surgeon, neurologist, cardiologist, gastroenterologist, pulmonologist, or psychiatrist. Soon after talking with Norm, I resolved to share the truth about John's illness with a few select people beyond my parents, Robert, and Nancy, including two close college friends. One, a gay man and his lovely partner, immediately became "uncles" to my children, helping me do everything from feed and bathe them to building their labyrinthine Ikea bedroom set. The other, a former roommate whose brother had recently died of AIDS, had a knack for showing up with her boyfriend at the very moment when I'd lost it, plying me with greasy potato chips in front of the TV or taking Caroline for a swim at her condo's health club. They knew AIDS, these folks, and had the haunted eyes to prove it. I also told my trusty running posse, who quickly took charge of my children's daily routines. Every weekday morning, one or the other would retrieve Caroline for the Y and either deposit her back home afterward or include her in their plans for the day. If anyone asked about the nature of John's illness, the party line was "viral encephalitis." Within days, the shelves of mosquito repellent and tall rubber boots at our local hardware store were picked clean.

At our corner drugstore, I sweated bullets every time I refilled John's prescription for AZT, the new AIDS drug. Had that ornery pharmacist shared the news with the liquor store guy next door, and he with the bagel man? "You know that red-headed guy who used to carry his little blond daughter on his shoulders every Saturday morning? Yeah, the guy with the chatty wife who was just pregnant—yeah, that guy—*he* has AIDS? That guy? He's *gay*?" When I walked down the street with my stroller, was I imagining their stares? Was I imagining that after seeing us, they quickly crossed the street? A heavy, dark cloud of stigma lurked outside our apartment walls.

Whenever I had time to spare at home, I plowed through the mountain of unopened bills toppling from the kitchen table onto the floor. Not only were there thick envelopes from doctors and insurers, there were the regular bills John managed: mortgage, gas, electric, his outstanding business school loan, not to mention those for our condo building, as I'd forgotten he was its president. John, meanwhile, padded around our apartment from bed to couch to bed again, and occasionally to the refrigerator, a cigarette dangling from his mouth.

Not long after my energizing meeting with Norm, I decided to try to shake John out of his stupor by asking for help. I went to him, lying on the bed watching TV, and asked if he would join me to look at the bills. He struggled up, put on his stylish wire-rimmed glasses, and padded after me to the dining table.

I placed our mortgage bill in front of him. "What about this one? Should I continue to pay it monthly, at this rate? What else should I know about it?" Silence.

I dug through the pile for his Harvard Business School loan statement. "How about this one? You don't have much more to pay, and the interest is high. We have enough to pay it off. Should I do it? And what about this trash bill for the building?"

John stared at me, his big blue eyes expressionless behind filthy lenses. I waited for him to say something, anything. Finally, he slurred, "I don't know, Maggie. I just don't know." He shook his head slightly, took a long drag of his cigarette, and limped back to the bedroom.

So this was how it was going to be, I realized. My partner in all things was gone; I was now on my own. It was going to be grim. But I was also the mother of two small children: grim wasn't in my job description. It was summer, and the kids needed sun and fresh air. Then again, where? We couldn't exactly go to the nearby park. Too many questions. Plus, who would watch John? So when Robert and his wife, Nancy, offered us their Connecticut house by the Long Island Sound for a few days, it seemed like the perfect solution. I packed up John, his pills, the babies, everyone's diapers, and off we went.

We left early enough to avoid Saturday morning traffic and arrived before lunch. I set up the playpen and portable crib, fed John and Caroline on the back deck, then nursed Dan and placed him down, drowsy, on his blanket. John dozed in an Adirondack chair, his cigarette burning down in an ashtray on its arm. I sat, too, for a minute, the sun on my face, a lovely breeze cooling my skin. Nice. I let myself drift off, then woke with a start. Where was I? Oh, right. Robert's house. There was Dan on the blanket, John in the chair, and...my eyes darted around the deck and football-field-sized lawn. Caroline. Where was Caroline? I ran inside, calling for her as I rushed through the living room, kitchen, dining room, den. I tore upstairs and heard plaintive whimpering from behind the bathroom door. "Mommy... help! Mommy...I can't get out!"

"Hold on, honey," I implored, jiggling the lock. I coached my little girl to try turning the knob one way, then the other, while from an open window I could hear Dan wailing. "John, can you help the baby?" I yelled out the window. Finally some combination of turning and jiggling worked and Caroline flew into my arms. I carried her, sobbing, down to the deck, where Dan was on his blanket, red-faced, wet, and miserable. John hadn't moved, his cigarette dangling from his mouth almost entirely burned down, ashes wafting to his chest. "John!" I said. "The baby!" John shifted his gaze from the baby to me, looking quizzical. Was I speaking Greek?

I suddenly did not want to be, for one more minute, in someone else's house in a town where I knew no one, taking care of a desperately sick man with a disease no one could know about, with a toddler and newborn infant in tow. Had I lost my mind? Cursing and stomping, I tore apart the portable crib and playpen I'd so meticulously constructed hours before, and hurled them into the trunk of the car. John sat motionless and expressionless, his swollen ankles casually crossed. My two babies were wailing. In what felt like record time, I loaded the car, strapped everyone in, and zoomed back to our hot Hoboken apartment.

The next weekend, I asked Robert and Nancy if they would watch John while I whisked the kids away, this time to visit my parents in Philadelphia. It was just one of many times during John's illness that my brother- and sister-in-law would host him at their home, where they, along with their babysitter, would unflinchingly clean and diaper him. It didn't matter that he sometimes bled, putting Nancy, in the early months of pregnancy, and their one-year-old son at risk. Their house was an absolute no-fear zone.

I packed the kids, their toys, and their gear up once again, and two hours later felt my spine relax as I pulled into the familiar driveway. I turned around to unstrap the sleeping kids from their car seats. As I unclicked Dan's restraint, a rush of heat emanated from his slack little body. I felt his forehead. The kid was burning up—just like John had been!

"Dad!" I yelled, rushing my infant entourage through the front door.

Mom scurried out of the kitchen, drying her hands; my dad appeared on the upstairs landing in his undershorts, newspaper and glasses in hand, and hurried down. "Mag—what is it?"

"Dan's sick!" I cried.

My father placed his tennis-callused palm on Dan's forehead and winced. I knew he was thinking what I was: My AIDS test had been wrong. It had to have been wrong.

It was eight-thirty at night and we had to find a doctor. My father unearthed a copy of the Yellow Pages and frantically thumbed through its thin grease-stained sheets until he found a pediatrician around the corner. We called, and he agreed to open up his office and give Dan a look.

Dr. Irwin Jacobs was a thin, unkempt, elderly man whose makeshift office, tacked onto his garage, made his medical licensure seem questionable. Feeling it necessary under the circumstances, I stammered out the fact that Dan's father had been recently diagnosed with AIDS. He practically dropped Dan on the hard linoleum floor in his haste to grab the phone and call the hospital to admit my feverish son, no doubt to get him—no, all of us, the whole AIDS-related kit and caboodle—out of his office and out of his life.

My dad and I hightailed it out to the car, the hot baby flopping on my breast. My father's anger was palpable; I knew he wanted to slug the guy, too. But I also knew that Dr. Jacobs wasn't the only one who felt that way. It was the world.

We zoomed onto Roosevelt Boulevard to St. Christopher's Hospital for Children, where they put Dan in a huge, metal, cagelike crib and tapped his tiny spine for bacterial sepsis and viruses, including HIV.

I spent that night sitting in a hard metal chair next to my baby's cold metal crib, contemplating the odds of my AIDS test being wrong. If we were all sick, I'd have to find a way to kill us. Better instant death than to watch my innocent children wasting away, battling debilitating illness and stigma. I didn't want to go that way, either. But how? Pills. Or drowning. No, pills. Could babies take pills? I wasn't sure. Drowning, then. "Please, no more," I cried. "Please."

The next morning, a bleary-eyed intern poked his head in and woke me, slumped in the chair. "Mrs. Andrew, your son has an ear infection," he reported, grinning. "That's all. An ear infection!" I laughed and hugged him hard, nearly breaking his glasses. Was I imagining the relief I also saw on his face? Just an ear infection! The petrifying absurdity of it all.

I raced down the hall to the pay phone and called my parents, sharing the exhilarating news, then realized I was starving. I hadn't eaten in…days? In the cafeteria, I devoured tuna salad swimming in Thousand Island dressing and a soggy, gigantic wedge of coconut cream pie. It was one of the best meals of my life.

A few hours later, my dad and I triumphantly returned home with a medicated, bright-eyed, chipper Dan. My mother handed me a message from Laura Popper, our trusted pediatrician in New York, whom the hospital had contacted. I dialed her back.

"You wanted to jump off the roof these past twenty-four

hours, didn't you?" she answered, ignoring the customary hello. A lanky, take-no-prisoners woman who favored red cowboy boots and had spent her girlhood crusading for racial equality, Dr. Popper was one of my New York heroes, always accessible for wise counsel. "You don't have AIDS, Maggie. None of you do. You know that, right?"

It would take years of Dr. Popper's calm reassurances, not to mention—when she could no longer take my insistence upon it—a definitive retesting of my kids for me to accept that we weren't sick. But for that one brief, relieved, shining moment, I believed her. We did not have AIDS.

Back in Hoboken, I dramatically recounted Dan's illness to his father. I might as well have been telling John his toast was ready. He sat and smoked. It was then I knew I'd had enough. Something had to give.

It wasn't only John's dazed unresponsiveness. He left half-smoked cigarettes burning all over the place, often perilously close to the baby. We lived among bleeding sores, secretions, soiled diapers. With John surviving far beyond the projected two weeks, the three flights of stairs up to our apartment and the multiplying trips to Manhattan doctors had become untenable. Meanwhile, my weight was plummeting. My hair was falling out, my gums bleeding, my skin cracking, my nights sleepless. Mercifully, help was on its way. Robert offered to put John up in his Manhattan pied-à-terre, located a few short blocks from Mount Sinai hospital and John's many doctors.

The apartment saved us. John had an escape from my withering anger and enforced sequestering, and, thanks to help from the *Journal*, round-the-clock attendants to serve his every need.

Colleagues and friends visited frequently for lunch, walks in the park, dinners at neighborhood restaurants. Their conversations revolved around the day's news, or the latest episode of *Twin Peaks*, politely avoiding loaded questions I constantly faced about his sexual orientation and how he contracted the disease. Robert shot up frequently from his midtown office, occasionally spending the night, and Nancy traveled down from Connecticut to bring supplies or have a meal with John, her baby in tow. Shortly after moving to the apartment, John's fog began to lift. Within weeks, the *Journal* began sending him editing work by courier. A few weeks after that, they began sending a limousine to bring him down to the office, along with his daily attendant, Charles Dunphey.

Charles was a slim, spritely, even-tempered man from Jamaica, never without a smile and attuned to everyone's needs. When I brought the kids to the apartment, Charles got down on the carpet and played Lego. He made me cups of tea. At Christmas, he bought and decorated a small tree for John and the kids. And when he diapered John, he threw diapering Dan into the deal, no charge. Best of all, Charles provided John with pot. Decades before San Francisco's storefront medicinal marijuana dispensaries, Charles was quietly dispensing to the AIDS patients he cared for.

When the weather was nice, Charles took John out for walks in nearby Carl Schurz Park. John had to have enjoyed placid Charles as a walking companion so much more than he did me, my one hand steering Caroline ahead, the other readjusting Dan in his Snuggli while also struggling to assist their father up and down steep curbs and steps, and across streets before the lights changed. More than once he fell, the stalled traffic honking angrily. I'd hurriedly help him up, feeling pity but also anger and shame as people stopped and stared. Could they tell that John, so young and so sick with "that look," had AIDS? I worried even more that they'd think I was his wife or his sister. Better his sister. Worst of all, John never said a word on these walks.

But for Charles—kind, chill Charles—John was, undoubtedly, just one more young, sick, dying man he tenderly nursed until death. For John, Charles had all the patience in the world. John talked to Charles, and Charles talked to me. We had our own little game of telephone. Charles loved being able to gussy John up and take him to work, mostly because John liked so much to go. He delighted in squeezing John—portly for the first time in his life, thanks to the drugs and sedentary lifestyle—into his Italian suits, making him feel dapper again. Then they'd be chauffered down to the World Financial Center in the *Journal*'s shiny black sedan. Charles loved the look of pride on John's face as they made their way down the hall to his corner office, everyone calling out, "Good to see you, Andrew!"

Then one day, one of John's scabs broke at the office and bled liberally on his desk, as well as on the reporter's work he'd been editing. The reporter scurried out of John's office and Charles was asked to take John home shortly after. Charles tried to explain the situation to John on the way home, but John became argumentative and angry, claiming that he "just didn't understand."

The next day, one of the *Journal*'s top editors contacted me. He felt terrible about what had happened and thought it best for everyone if John worked from home instead.

John refused to understand why this debacle had even occurred. From the moment of his diagnosis, he never once mentioned or acknowledged that he had AIDS. The closet was where he would steadfastly remain. Four times during the course of his illness, John was hospitalized for infections and placed in the hospital's AIDS cluster. And every single time, he demanded to be relocated. "I don't belong here," he'd say.

Just as the apartment gave John a life separate from me, it gave me one separate from him. Without John, I had a chance to mother my two small children. And just as it allowed John a refuge from the prying eyes and flying rumors of our Hoboken neighborhood, it gave me periodic breaks from them, too.

Every weekend, I packed up the kids, their portable cribs and Steiff toys, and we headed into Manhattan to visit their father. By now, Dan was beginning to lift his head up off his blankie and gurgle and make faces, and John would tickle him, then doze off with Dan in his lap. Caroline and I serial-watched episodes of the age-inappropriate *Degrassi Junior High* on television. For dinner, we ordered pizza, or burgers and fries from a nearby diner. It became routine to "go see Daddy." Will I ever forget the questioning stares and whispers from the posh Upper East Side neighbors ("What's wrong with him, so young?") as the four of us struggled back from our brief walks, me juggling greasy takeout while shifting Dan's weight in the Snuggli and helping John maneuver his cane, Caroline trailing crankily behind, as I attempted to usher us through the apartment building's heavy revolving doors?

When Halloween came along, I took the kids—Caroline dressed as a pumpkin in bright orange felt, Dan zipped into a watermelon suit—to show John their costumes. He just about managed a smile.

Sometimes, when a friend offered to take the kids for the weekend, I would visit John alone. Gone were the days of affectionate endearments and hot sex; my time with him was now spent making sure he was fed, helping him shower and dress, and tidying the apartment. I no longer saw myself as his wife or lover. Now I was one of his helpers, perhaps his chief helper. Over the months, I finally gave up hoping to hear words of apology, remorse, or explanation. If John talked, it was mostly about work, or friends who had visited. I learned to keep it light. Once I shared a problem Caroline was having at preschool, and in response, he pantomimed playing the violin. I stormed out of the room. But then, he was dying. In the scheme of things, what were a preschooler's problems? Or mine?

During one such weekend, we were sitting next to each other on the apartment's tufted loveseat. John sidled closer, resting his head on my shoulder, and sighed. I let myself rest my head on his. We sat like that for a while. We were a married couple, perched there together in Robert's high-rise pied-à-terre, but we were not remotely the same people who had wed each other on that exuberant summer day in 1986. We were people who, in a flash, had lost each other and everything we had together. And at that moment, we both knew it. It was the saddest moment of his illness, if not our entire union.

Over the months, as John's health declined, I set aside my anger and tried passionately to keep him alive. Each time he was hospitalized, I kept a bedside vigil, hiring expert nursing care to give him at least one more day. This most unlucky of men would not, it seemed, live to see thirty-seven. He would not live to see his son's first birthday. The stigma-free zone of Robert's apartment and, certainly, of the hospital freed me to feel sad for John, for us, for what could have been.

Back in Hoboken, it was another story. There, John's outline remained, like a chalk outline after a murder, marked with big, angry question marks. Where was he? Where did he go? Was he alive or dead? What did he really have? People wouldn't stop asking. I strived to keep myself and my two sunny, cherubic blonds in sync with the "Mommy 'n' Me" activities around town, smiling woodenly and lying through my teeth. The less I said, the better. I'd hustle us out of puppet shows before everyone else to avoid the need to chat. "What a bitch," people whispered. "What's wrong with her?" Why, I wouldn't even take their advice when they recommended neurologists! It *was* a brain tumor, wasn't it? Or didn't somebody say encephalitis, or was that meningitis? I was confounding—people didn't get me, were put off. John and his disease were a mystery, and we were selfish for not sharing. If they'd have known, they might have understood. Or, some people might have. It was agonizing trying to decide whom.

Often, I'd bump into someone at the supermarket, perhaps a woman I'd met at a party the year before. "I heard your husband was sick," she'd say. "What's wrong with him?" If she was an artist, or maybe politically liberal, I might take a chance and reveal that John had AIDS. "Is he gay, or a drug addict?" she might then ask. And, "How is it you don't have it—are you sure?" and "You have kids, so you must have had sex together. How can you not be sick?" Or she might zero in on the subject of John being gay: "Did you know?" I always struggled not to reply, "Oh sure, I knew. He told me he was gay on our first date!" Worst of all, she might say, "Aren't you angry? *I* would be."

Yes, I was angry. Angry with John, and angry that I couldn't tell the truth without fielding these incessant questions, prying into every nook and cranny of my marriage and sex life. In my better moments, I realized that I, too, might ask these questions if someone's husband had AIDS. But my fury and panic blinded me. Why couldn't they just stop asking? When I couldn't take any more, I decided once again, as my father and Robert had advised, not to tell anyone...anything. To close up shop. I retreated back inside. I called no one except my running circle; all play-dates with anyone else's kids ceased. The phone stopped ringing. I skipped the playground, and attended no school events unless flanked by my confidants.

Stuck inside our four walls, my anger roiled. Where to put it? Staggering with sleep deprivation, I exploded at whoever was around—usually my parents, so fraught with worry they were practically living with us. In response, my dad would counsel, "Don't get bitter, Mag, it's the worst thing you can be." He'd then quote Henry Ford II, who, when nailed on drunk driving charges, purportedly said, "Never complain, never explain." There had to be a more inspiring role model, but at least my dad was trying.

There wasn't any more sympathy from my mother, with her steely positive resolve and allegiance to my father in all things. Robert and Nancy, wrestling with their grief privately, were supportive in every way possible but didn't talk to me about

John much beyond the practical. Likely they couldn't; fury was shooting off me in hot sparks. For a sounding board, I had to look elsewhere.

Fortunately, I didn't have to go far. Once John moved to the apartment, I went back to running nearly every weekday morning with my Y gang and regularly poured my heart out. As we set out on our run, one or another would ask, "How is he?" In response to each story I shared, no matter how horrific—John's fall in the street, his bleeding at work, his latest diagnosis—there was always an empathetic response, practical solution, or juicy piece of gossip to make us all chortle. These women were my eyes and ears, keeping me abreast of what people were saying, not to mention of my kids' progress at swimming lessons and behavior on playdates. As we jogged down the road, I felt shielded by them. Among us was Lucia, an Episcopal minister whose spiritual guidance pulled me more than once from despair. In many ways, this daily run became my church.

There were other saviors in my midst, too. Living in the condo downstairs were a young divorcée, Mary Ellen Atkinson, her mother, Elvira Diaz (known to us as "the Abuela"), and Mary Ellen's three kids, Rachel, Patrick, and Michelle. John had been a hot ticket with them for his ability to help solve complex algebra problems in a pinch—often the night before a big test. The two girls regularly watched our kids anyway, but when John became ill, Mary Ellen set up a "don't ask, don't tell," round-the-clock babysitting service. There are more pictures of Dan as a baby with the Abuela than with me. Two floors down, at street level, was a specialty food store owned by a lapsed priest, Ray, whose father, Gabe, sliced deli meat while crooning, "I love you more today than yesterday (but not as much as tomorrow)," from a hit song of the late 1960s. I often absconded to Ray's for tea, sympathy, and a fresh baked roll. "Don't ask, don't tell" was his credo, too.

And then there was Susan. Like the Y running moms, she frequently brought casseroles and took the kids when I had to be in the city, but she went further, taking control of my mountains of medical bills and insurance claims, organizing, color-coding, and filing them. When I needed to visit my parents with the kids in Philadelphia, she'd come along and help. Wellesley educated, resourceful, and unceasingly calm, Susan became my right hand when I had barely a leg to stand on. I loved my running moms, but I *needed* Susan.

That is, until one cold, rainy Friday in early November, three months after John had moved to the apartment. With no Y child care available on Fridays, it had become the one day I gave us all a break from the rushed morning routine. With the weather forecast gloomy, I decided we'd cozily stay in and amuse ourselves. I fed and bathed the kids, then treated myself to a long, hot shower.

Catching a glimpse of myself in the mirror over the sink, I noticed that I was markedly slimmer. I had hipbones—every zaftig Jewish girl's dream. I'd barely had time to eat, and for the first time in my weight-obsessed life, I had no appetite. I vowed to cook something nutritious for lunch. Yes, that's what I'd do. After this hot shower, I'd have a hot lunch. Begin to take better care of myself.

Relaxed and refreshed, I settled down on the couch to watch the kids. Dan dozed in his bouncy seat; Caroline was engrossed in a one-way conversation with Barbie. I flipped through one of the unread *New Yorker* magazines piling up on the table. Friends had recently taken up a collection to provide me with a monthly cleaning service, and the house smelled, comfortingly, of Pledge. I called Charles to check in. He reported their daily walk to the park had been aborted by rain, and also that he'd discovered John trying to shower with his clothes on.

We shared a wry chuckle, but it wasn't funny. My once competent, graceful, beyond brilliant John couldn't finish sentences, toppled over in the street, and forgot to undress before bathing. I arranged to relieve Charles early the next morning, then hung up and looked at the kids again. At least we had our lives ahead of us. At least we had that.

The door buzzer sounded.

I wasn't expecting anyone. Maybe it was one of my running buddies dropping by. Or Susan? I went to the intercom by the door. "Who is it?"

"It's DYFS, Mrs. Andrew," a woman's voice garbled back.

"Die-what?"

"The Division of Youth and Family Services," the voice repeated. "May I come up?"

What, now? I hesitated. With AIDS in the house—even the specter of AIDS—you had to be careful. Government agencies could only spell trouble. But what could I do? "Okay," I said, buzzing her in.

A few minutes later, I opened the condo door to a wet, pleasant looking young woman with slightly smeared mascara. She introduced herself as Carrie Canaday, a state-employed social worker. While removing her soaked slicker, she let her eyes alight on each child, then turned to me to report she was following up on an anonymous report of child abuse. Could I please remove my children's diapers?

"Somebody called to report child abuse here?" I asked, incredulous. "Do you know that my husband, the father of these children, has AIDS?"

The young woman looked stunned. "No," she said. "Mrs. Andrew, I did *not* know that. I'm so sorry. Is he here somewhere?"

I explained that John now lived in the city, and what had happened since July. I was shaking. Was I about to lose my kids, the only good thing left in my sorry life?

"Who would do such a thing?" I asked.

"Ma'am, it's anonymous—we can't say," she responded. Then, sympathetically, she said, "Mrs. Andrew, looking at your kids and your home, I see you have things together here. But I still need to look under those diapers. Could you please remove them?"

"What kind of abuse is this?" I pressed.

She looked at me and said nothing.

"Sexual," I confirmed.

She nodded.

Panic threatened to choke me. "You're not going to take my kids away, are you?" I cried. "Don't take my kids away—please!"

She said nothing.

"Which kid?" I persisted, horrified.

"Both," she said.

As if in slow motion, I walked over to my son dozing in his little seat, picked him up, untaped his blue pampers with its decorative band of colorful trucks, and laid him out on the dining room table. The social worker inspected him closely, back and front, and gave me the okay to return him to his seat.

Next was Caroline, who by now had abandoned her doll to pad over and see what was happening. On the verge of three, she'd been wearing mostly underpants. I gently pulled her toward me and lowered their elastic waistband, explaining that the lady just had to look at her quickly.

Ms. Canaday kneeled down, looked Caroline over, and gave me permission to pull up her Carters. "Go play now, honey," she told her.

"Mrs. Andrew, I'm sorry I had to come here today and do this," she said. "I'm also sorry about what happened to your husband. I do have to file a report, but I saw nothing here in the way of abuse and will recommend that this case be closed."

I thanked her profusely, showed her out, and rushed to call Susan. She'd know just what to do about this. Susan could always be depended on for a split-second, surefooted plan of defense.

"Hello," Susan answered.

"Susan!" Then, in a rush: "Oh, my God, you'll never guess what's happened. The Division of Youth and Family Services just came—apparently somebody anonymously reported me for child abuse!"

Susan's response to this explosive bit of news was as calm as always. "Wow. That's too bad," she said. "But look, I have to take Jessie out somewhere—can I call you back?"

"Sure," I said. *Click.*

Who else should I call? I dialed Dr. Popper.

"I know who did this to you," she said immediately.

"You do?"

"Yes, that friend of yours—Susan."

Dr. Popper said that Susan had called her earlier that week to say she'd seen marks on Caroline, and to ask if she thought I was abusing her. "I told her I checked Caroline and Dan frequently and had never seen any kind of marks. I told her I thought you were doing an amazing job, and don't have the strength to pick out toilet paper let alone abuse anyone. I told her I could not, and would not, support her accusation.

"I didn't tell you she called," she continued, "because I didn't want to scare you. I also didn't think she'd do anything more than call me. Clearly I was wrong. Stay away from her."

After I hung up with Dr. Popper, I sprang into action, contacting the Y child-care teachers and the local church preschool teacher requesting they send letters to the DYFS endorsing me as a parent. I also asked this of Lucia and my friend Judy, a children's publishing executive who served on several child welfare boards and took my kids on the weekends I visited John.

In early January, I received a letter from the DYFS:

Dear Ms. Maggie Kneip,
Re: Caroline and Daniel

We have completed our assessment/investigation in regard to the referral received on the above mentioned child(ren). Since at this time no need for services is indicated and you have not requested continued services, we will be terminating our agency's involvement effective 1/11/91. Thank you for your help and cooperation during our recent contacts. If, in the future, you should have need of our services, please feel free to contact our agency.

At the bottom of the letter, Ms. Canaday had scrawled: "Sorry for the 'upsetness' this caused but under the law the Division is mandated to investigate all allegations of abuse. It appears your children are very well cared for and lucky to have you as a mom. Sincerely, C.C."

Susan never did call me back. In fact, we never spoke again. Why did she do it? Was it to sever herself from any relationship with me? To remove my children from an "AIDS house"? To rescue them from something she fantasized was happening? The whole episode became one more dirty, dark secret I kept to myself. After that cold November day, I got tougher. If people feared me, I now also feared them.

As John's mysterious illness wore on, the stress on our family mounted and Caroline's little face became progressively darker. At school, she began regularly bolting out of class crying. Her teachers were jittery, confounded about what to do. I did everything short of buying her a pony to keep things light. Eventually, I sought the advice of a child psychologist who in the course of our treatment referred me to an AIDS support group for HIV-negative wives.

Until connecting with this unmerry little band, I had felt so alone: a straight woman whose husband was dying of AIDS. Everyone else it touched seemed male, and gay. Attending my first meeting, in the basement of an ivy-covered Greenwich Village church, was like coming home.

We were the wife of a convict, a septuagenarian grandmother, a B-52s roadie, and yours truly, a yuppie deer in the headlights. Each week we exchanged our personal horror stories, along with best practices for protecting our kids from the stigma of the disease. Our facilitators were hollow-eyed social workers caught up in the same predicament. "Protecting our kids is our first priority," they said. "Lie if you have to, and if they are old enough to understand why, teach your kids to lie as well. Almost no one out there really understands AIDS."

I turned thirty-five at Robert's tiny kitchenette table, both kids on my lap, Nancy setting out the plates, and a diapered John by my side, listing dangerously on his folding chair. We wore party hats, the whole motley crew—what the heck. I'd picked up a hot pink birthday cake from the corner supermarket and a box of candles, and before blowing them out, I wished hard that it would all be over soon.

By spring 1991, it was. In his final weeks, John's friends and family materialized from far and near. It was a poignant time of good-bye.

Except for John and me, that is.

For us, there was too much left unsaid.

Dear Maggie,

I wanted to tell you that one of these days, we will—
1. Sit in a white loft with high ceilings and drink Puerto Rican rum drinks
2. Be high in the Rockies
3. Kiss in the fog on the Golden Gate Bridge
4. Go on a juice fast
5. (your turn).

Love, John

Seven

I'm Maggie Kneip. I was John's wife.

*I think most of you here know that in losing John, I've lost the
best husband a girl could ever want. I've lost my best friend, too. But
I have also, like so many of you, lost my best editor—someone who,
with one kind but pointed remark, shake of his red head, or sidelong
glance, could silence or streamline me, when entirely appropriate.*

So began my eulogy of John at the New-York Historical
Society in New York City on Tuesday, March 27, 1991.
Looking back, it's hard to believe the person who wrote
those words could possibly be me. Then again, I was a young
woman whose husband had just died, reading words I'd hastily
thrown together to a blur of four hundred people. I couldn't say
what I really thought, though I'm quite sure I was conflicted as
to what exactly that was.

Of course, there were anger and betrayal. There were
trauma, heartbreak, and desolation. I was dazed and disoriented,
haunted by memories and unanswered questions. I found myself

calling out to John in the middle of the night, and to every young redheaded man on the street. Around that time, the actor David Caruso was becoming famous for his upcoming role in a TV show called *NYPD Blue*. Red hair, fit, impeccably dressed, mysterious and reserved—he was a dead ringer for John, and there he was, everywhere I turned, on what seemed to be every magazine cover.

And I couldn't say, that day, what killed John. Like the twelve other people speaking at that service, many of them America's most respected journalists, I couldn't say "AIDS."

Just after John died, Norman Pearlstine called me at home. In order to protect me and the children, he said, he'd contacted his counterpart at *The New York Times* to request the cause of John's death be omitted from his obituary. In the end, it read:

JOHN F. ANDREW
EDITOR, 36

John F. Andrew, an editor and former columnist with The Wall Street Journal, *died on Thursday at Mount Sinai Medical Center in Manhattan. He was 36 years old and lived in Hoboken, N.J. He died of lymphoma, said his brother, Robert, of Westport, Conn. Mr. Andrew, a graduate of Brown University and Harvard Business School, joined* The Wall Street Journal *as a reporter in Los Angeles in 1980. In addition to this brother, he is survived by his wife, Margaret Kneip; a daughter, Caroline; a son, Daniel; and his parents, Merle and Alice, of Bethesda, Maryland.*

Two columns away was an obituary for "Tomas Cabrera, Lawyer, 38, who'd died of AIDS, a family spokesman said." Such was the gross inequity of AIDS at that time; Mr. Cabrera was unmarried, and without children. I, a mother of two defenseless babies, was deeply in debt to Norm for his precautionary, protective act. Things were already hard enough for us in Hoboken—on the streets, in the playground, in the classroom—without a national newspaper broadcasting the news that my kids' father had died of AIDS.

Back at the New-York Historical Society, *Wall Street Journal* assistant manager Paul Steiger was praising John from the podium:

> *How to think about John? I suppose the easy comparison is as a Renaissance man—a Renaissance man of journalism. He was omni-competent, but it was much more than that, he was original and creative with everything he touched. But in trying to think of a template for John, I think not of the Renaissance, but of a couple of centuries later, the eighteenth century: this year is exactly the 200th anniversary of the death of Mozart. And like Mozart, John was blessed with huge talent. He accomplished great things in a life that was too short. I will miss him very much, but I will treasure the memory of having known him.*

I'd organized the service with Barney Calame, the *Journal's* assistant managing editor, who could often be found by John's side, and mine, during the course of John's illness. It was my job to select the program's speakers and create its order. Robert, so aggrieved by his brother's untimely death, wanted to close the program and did so, affectingly. Me, I spoke in the middle, where I could remain comfortably invisible.

At the service that day, as the quintessential Renaissance man's widow, I was in love all over again. But as the widow of the man with the disease that couldn't be named, I longed to find a hole somewhere and crawl in. When the auditorium was empty and everyone returned to their houses and jobs and lives and loves, there were only me, two small children, and our lives to rebuild.

By the year John died, 1991, AIDS had killed 157,637 mostly gay men in this country; 257,750 more had been diagnosed. A proud red AIDS ribbon began appearing on people's lapels, and a massive AIDS Memorial Quilt was being stitched, each square representing another person lost and mourned. Eight months later, the NBA star Magic Johnson, a married man, would go on national television to announce that he, too, had the virus.

Image after image began to appear on front pages and network news, of gay men who nursed each other and who prayed, fought, and protested, their tears illuminated in candlelight vigils. Like them, I'd lost my young lover to this disease, but there our similarities ended. They were out; I was a mother desperate to keep my husband's secrets in the closet. They were proud; I was ashamed. Part of me was dying to cry out, "We've lost someone to this horrible disease, too!"

I didn't dare.

A few weeks after the service, Robert called to see if I wanted to drive up to the family's ancestral plot in Meredith, New Hampshire, to bury John's ashes. It would be just Robert and me, putting John to rest in quiet dignity. Perfect. Except, I didn't want to go. Hadn't we just had a massive memorial service, followed by an impromptu shiva involving a dozen reporters showing up at my door with smoked fish platters from Zabar's? Since the memorial service, I'd felt depleted, barely able to get out of bed. I couldn't just spring up and go to New Hampshire. I'd have to find a babysitter, figure out how Caroline would get to school, rearrange playdates. And what about the kids' dinner?

The next thing I knew, I was sitting next to Robert in his blue Taurus, unseasonably clad in shorts, flip-flops, a tank top, and John's old windbreaker as we zoomed up to New Hampshire. Robert was at the wheel; John was in a box on the backseat. Dawn was breaking; we sleepily made small talk.

Meredith is a charming, historic little town on Lake Winnipesaukee where John spent the summers of his youth lolling around his grandparents' hillside farmhouse, with a spectacular view of the lake. The family had a long history intertwined with the town.

The wind whipped and cold rain drizzled as Robert carried the box over to a fresh hole prepared by the gravediggers. I was freezing, my flip-flops sliding across the wet, muddy earth. Robert laid John's ashes carefully in the ground, and then, to my surprise, began nearly wailing the classic Irish ballad "Danny Boy."

Oh Danny boy, the pipes, the pipes are calling
From glen to glen, and down the mountain side
The summer's gone, and all the flowers are dying
'tis you, 'tis you must go and I must bide.

As he sang, Robert closed his eyes; anguish flickered across the sad alabaster mask of his face. It was an intensely personal moment of grief, a moment in which he said good-bye to his baby brother with the fiery red hair. I stood next to him, astonished by the deep love and mourning flowing from him. Astonished, but not sad. Not sharing in Robert's profound grief. Not putting my arm around him in solidarity and comfort. I stood apart, detached, staring hard at the little box of John in the ground. I felt numb, holding fast to my denial. Since his diagnosis, I'd never been able to face the fact that John would die. Now I couldn't bear that he was gone. Even after all that had happened, I didn't want to be in a world without John Andrew.

Robert finished singing and stood over John's hole in the ground, then turned to me and almost violently pulled me into a crushing embrace. It was all I could do to hug back for dear life. If I felt anything that cold April day, it was sadness for Robert, standing alone at his little brother's grave, unleashing searing grief. Afterward, he and I silently went up the lane to his cousin's house for coffee and danish.

After that mournful day, Robert rarely spoke to me about John, except with regard to practical and financial concerns—especially those concerning Dan and Caroline, for whom, I was gratified to see, he felt no end of responsibility. Which is not to say, as Nancy later shared, that he didn't mourn his brother deeply and speak of him often to her, and to his sons. Just not to me. I came to understand that as close as Robert and I each were to John, we couldn't mourn him similarly, or together. Years later, I was to feel this same fissure of experience with my grown children.

Some months after John's internment, I ordered a slim granite headstone for his grave, with the inscription:

John F. Andrew
Devoted father
of
Caroline Alice
and
Daniel Kneip Andrew
and
Beloved husband
of Margaret Kneip
Born July 10, 1954
Washington, D.C.
Died March 21, 1991
New York City.
He lived a life that mattered.
We miss him.

I imagined the Concord, New Hampshire, stone cutters, as they chiseled this mawkish epitaph, musing, "What the...? Who *doesn't* live a life that matters?"

It was a line lifted from a eulogy at John's memorial, delivered by Lucia, the minister from my running group:

We know that John led a life that mattered, a life that, if you will, went for the gold, a life he poured out for others, for beliefs, for love. He led a life that went beyond comfort and safety, and he loved a woman who possesses the same quality. John enjoyed life, and he accomplished much. And his illness and his dying were hard, hard on him, hard on those he loved, and those who loved him. But now he is beyond, and with God, and reaching back to us, to us, his friends,

to his family, to his wife and children, and I believe that he might be
saying something like this to all of us here today. "Death is nothing
at all. I am only slipped away into the next room."

There was so much about my late husband's life I desperately
wanted to believe mattered. Night after night, he haunted my
dreams, sexy, smart, witty—and healthy. Like he once was. But
in the light of day, he'd died of AIDS; his life was now hidden in
shadows of secrecy and shame. What do you do with the memory of someone about whom you can't speak? The path of least
resistance was to also be dead: dead to any love I still felt for him,
dead to any memory or mention of him, dead to the open and
trusting person I once was. I needed to sever myself—and the
kids—from any association with his disease. To do that, I would
need to ditch John, too. Fast.

Dear Magski,

I think you are great, and how about that?

I am reading about Lenin and the dictatorship of the proletariat in Modern Times*—and then I take a break to watch the Academy Awards and the stretch limos rolling like tanks up the boulevard to the D. C. Pavilion, gray ones, black ones, white and silver—what would Lenin make of such an orgy of fantasy? Well, Vladimir? By the way, do you have any thoughts on Tim Hutton hooking up with Debra Winger?*

Your ever loving, spaced out, kind of shy, sexy, reserved, hot 'n' cold, mad about you,

John

Eight

After John's death, I rolled up my sleeves and cleared every visible trace of him from our condo. I was done with him and done with AIDS. His beautiful bespoke suits and designer shoes went off to Goodwill, his high-end ablutions into the trash, his stash of AZT flushed down the toilet. His baby pictures, awards, diplomas, newspaper clips, cards, and love letters were tossed into boxes and taped up tight for the kids.

But there was more stuff in John's office to pack up, which I was summoned to do a few weeks later. It would be my first time back at the *Journal* since that hot July day when I'd met with Norm Pearlstine. Now John was dead, and I was back, freshly blond and svelte (because who could eat?), heavily perfumed, and barely clad in a tiny white miniskirt and spiked heels, picking my way down the narrow aisle separating the reporters in their individual cubicles. It was a new me, dressed like the Farrah Fawcett look-alikes I'd always derided. Men noticed you when you looked like that, and I was desperate to be noticed.

One by one the reporters peered up from their screens to

watch me, wide-eyed, in deafening silence. Some managed to wanly call out, "Hi, Maggie!" Once in John's glass-enclosed corner office, a few strolled by, peering in while I tossed whatever I thought the kids might one day appreciate seeing into a box. This included a "Dow Jones All Points Bulletin" headlined "It's a Boy for John Andrew and Maggie Kneip," dated June 19, 1990, almost a year before. The last time I'd been happy.

Fighting back tears, I lugged the unwieldy box down the escalator and out to the PATH train, but once on it, the urge to cry ebbed. Balancing it on my nearly bare lap, I opened the copy of the *Journal* I'd pilfered from the office and willed myself not to think about anything but what I would make the kids for dinner.

"Whaddya doin'? Movin'?" barked the guy across from me. He was young and nice looking, with a nervously jiggling leg.

"What?" I answered, jolted from my reverie. "Oh…no. My husband died, and I cleaned out his office."

Loss had reduced my once confident, effusive voice to that of an injured bird. Some men loved that, I knew. He crossed the aisle to talk with me, then asked me out for a drink. Later that week, we slept together. Vinnie was ten years younger, Italian, a hard-charging salesman, an ex–college athlete who took his dinners nightly in the local sports bar. I'd sneak out to see him whenever I could get a babysitter. After several months, Vinnie got tired of this arrangement—and as he showed no interest in my kids, so did I. Terry was next, also a salesman, also a sports fan, also Italian. He actually liked to take my kids to the zoo—that is, when he didn't have a date with Jackie, Nancy, or Lisa.

Vinnie and Terry weren't going to replace John, and that was fine. It didn't take a PhD from Brown to know that I liked them because they were so different. In the year after John's death, I was desolate, shattered by loss, desperate to feel alive again. They were young, virile, and vibrantly healthy. Both men restored my interest in sex, making me feel desirable and beautiful in that trussed up, lip-glossed way I needed most. It was intoxicating to be wanted again.

At thirty-five, with two kids and no interest in a sparkling ring or dream home, I was the perfect date. Both Vinnie and Terry knew what killed my husband, but they weren't afraid of sleeping with me or averse to using condoms. This made them unusual. Many others were afraid to touch me. One particularly memorable blind date was with a film director named Tony. I'd arrived at the Soho restaurant early and ordered a vodka martini to calm myself, my hand shaking so hard that I splashed the drink all over my jeans. When Tony arrived, the first thing he said to me, chortling, was, "Just my luck! I have a blind date with a woman whose husband died of AIDS!" A real comedian. The check couldn't come fast enough.

Meanwhile, the reality of our financial situation was becoming increasingly clear: I needed a job. There were our mortgage, utilities, car payment, home and car insurance, and John's unpaid business school loan. We had the life insurance, some stocks, the lakefront property in New Hampshire, and a halfhearted promise of eventual support for college coming from Merle, but how to support the children until then? When my friend Judy offered me a job at her publishing company making author videos and licensing deals for kids' books with movie companies, I jumped at the chance. I was soon flying frequently to Los Angeles, the kids settled in with our new live-in nanny, who hailed from

Ireland but, as luck would have it, was sent from heaven.

With my available free nights waning, so did my dalliances with Vinnie and Terry. And as the two-year anniversary of John's death approached, I came to my senses, realizing that finding a suitable replacement father for my two babies was the most important thing. I asked my secretary if she knew anyone who fit the bill. She knew Dave.

As soon as I met Dave, I was struck by how very different he was from John. Although nice looking, a Georgetown graduate, and a voiceover talent agent, Dave was a "what you see is what you get" kind of guy. For him, stars were nothing more than exploding balls of hydrogen in the sky. He wore t-shirts with stretched-out necks and ill-fitting jeans, and said things like, "You're darn tootin'!" and "Coolicious, partner!" He lived alone in a dingy Chelsea rental, had been engaged once—or was it twice?—and spent a fair amount of time with ambitious, down-at-the-heel actresses. He had a mangy cat and, for my taste, drank a little too much.

Then again, Dave was single. He'd been an altar boy. He'd even been an Eagle Scout. And though I'd certainly been wrong before, I could tell he was straight. It was also hard to imagine someone who said "Jesus Christmas!" cheating on me. Plus, there were my aging parents and disabled brother to worry about, the car's oil and tires to change, dinner parties where I didn't want to be the odd woman out, and my lonely bed at night.

Best of all, Dave loved spending time with my kids. He loved it even more than spending time with me. He read them every book I brought home from work, from *Charlotte's Web* to

Watership Down, using a different voice for each character. He took them canoeing on the Delaware River. He taught them to ride bikes. He taught them to ski. He skipped down the street, holding their hands. He liked mint chocolate chip ice cream even more than they did. He got them a puppy. At Dan's third birthday party, only a few weeks after we started dating, Dave clambered all over the jungle gym with the little ones in his khaki business suit, quickly becoming the life of the party. Nancy pulled me aside and asked, "Where did you find him? Wow. Not bad, Maggie."

Dave was a crack mimic, a modern-day vaudevillian, a cheerful, "*no problema*" kind of guy. When you were around him, you pretty much had to be happy. After his predecessor, happy would do just fine. I could take everything but the drinking and the cat. The first he stopped cold, the second he pawned off. Oh, and the actresses moved on. To my surprise, Dave was a keeper.

Two years after John died, I had a boyfriend and a job. I was putting my life—our lives—back together again. Or so I told myself. In reality, people still crossed the street as I approached. Friends I'd once trusted continued to turn tail. That summer, I took the kids up to Vermont, to John's cousins' annual lakeside picnic. When we arrived, the hosts refused to shake my hand and recoiled from touching either child. I drove back to New Jersey late that night in a torrential rainstorm, cursing them, cursing John, cursing the toxic stain he'd left behind.

That summer, I received a letter from Caroline's private school indicating that she would not be moved up with her class to first grade. Though she had been reviewed as precocious ("off the charts" was how they'd put it), her teacher had struggled to handle her "transitional" home situation. I immediately scheduled a meeting with the school's director, who responded to my frantic questions with only vague generalities. "It's just a feeling we have," she said. "She's not ready."

I walked home fuming at her insensitivity, furious that Caroline would lose the familiarity of her friends moving up to the next grade. As I waited at a crosswalk, my blood boiling, I heard my name being called. It was a parent from Caroline's class, a mother from whom I always sensed a whiff of empathy.

"Maggie!" she called, flagging me down from across the street. "Hold on a minute, will you?"

"Helen," I said, and then spilled. "I'm so mad! I just got out of a meeting with Dr. Sussman. They're not moving Caroline up with Mark and the others next year." We both knew Caroline was farther ahead at school than Helen's son, Mark, not to mention most of the kids in the class. Something was up.

"Maggie, listen," she said, looking around and taking a step closer. "We had a parents' committee meeting last Monday. I don't know if you've heard about this, but someone suggested we take a vote to see if anyone felt...well, if people thought it was safe to send our kids to school with yours."

The traffic and noise of our town's main street suddenly fell away. Had I heard her right? I stared at Helen, who looked down. I'd heard right.

"Thanks for telling me," I said. "Who wanted the vote?"

Helen hesitated. "Beth."

Beth. Beth was a velvet-voiced woman who barely gave me the time of day—and was a close friend of Susan's. Was this some sort of witch hunt?

With that, I was done with hip, happening Hoboken, the scene of the crime. I put the condo up for sale and, through my children's publishing job, found a progressive public school in New York City that welcomed my kids with open arms, AIDS or no AIDS. I packed up and moved us all—Dave, too—into a two-bedroom rental apartment on the Upper East Side, one block from the school. It was a new start, a fresh beginning.

One afternoon at work, I got a call from Caroline's new first grade teacher, Layne. Earlier that day, Layne had read aloud to the class a book entitled *Daddy and Me*, by Jeanne Moutoussamy-Ashe, the widow of tennis star Arthur Ashe. Ashe had died of AIDS a short time after John, and the book was meant to memorialize him for their daughter. In the ensuing class discussion, Caroline had shot up her dimpled hand. "My dad died of AIDS, too," she'd announced.

My hand tightened on the receiver. Would we have to find yet another school? "We need to find another way for Caroline to say that," was all Layne gently suggested.

That evening, I pulled my five-year-old daughter onto my lap and asked her to pinky-swear that, when asked how her father had died, she'd say, "I don't want to talk about it," or if pressed further, "Cancer." Never, under any circumstances, should she say AIDS. Talk about a "bad" four-letter word.

In the end, the Manhattan New School, P.S. 290, provided us no end of restorative support and compassion, not to mention quality education. But eventually, Caroline hit fifth grade, the end of the line. We were also bursting the seams of our tiny two-bedroom apartment, where my near-adolescent daughter and her brother shared a room, and it was looking like we might soon have to take in my parents, now in varying states of decline. We began spending weekends strapped into our Honda Civic, the kids whining in the back as we scoured the suburbs of Lower Westchester and Northern Jersey for affordable houses in good school systems.

By this time I was director of publicity at a children's book publisher, and one day a woman strolled into my office to interview for a freelance assignment. She wore ripped jeans, an oversize oxford button-down shirt, muddy riding boots, bracelets she'd woven herself, and vibrant beads strung by women in Zimbabwe. Though it was November, she was sun-kissed. I was wearing one of the three nearly identical black pantsuits that comprised my office wardrobe, chunky costume jewelry from Loehmann's, and a blouse with a big coffee stain. I wanted to be her.

Like me, Jo was blond, blue-eyed, and Jewish, with a build like a Tyrolean hiker and a mouth like Sarah Silverman. Within seconds, we were *mano a mano* on comedic monologues. She was married to Drew, a television producer nearly ten years her senior and twice divorced. They had two children the same age as mine, whom she was staying home to raise and who, she said, were she not hired for this freelance gig, would drive her *meshugge*.

I felt instantly comfortable with this woman, so like me yet so much more alive. I went ahead and told her my own husband had died. "Of AIDS," I added impulsively, watching for her reaction.

Surprisingly, she didn't next inquire, "Was he gay?" Nor did she ask, "Do you have it?," "Are you sure your kids don't?," or "How could you not have it? You slept with him, didn't you?"

No. What Jo said was, "I'm sorry. That must be so tough."
And then, "Do you know how I can kill mine?"

It wasn't long before I, Dave, and the kids were spending almost every weekend at Jo's ranch house in Westport, Connecticut, where our kids somersaulted on the backyard trampoline and Jo made great mojitos and even better jokes about everyone and everything. No one was spared, not even John. When I told her that he had once sewn his own pair of pants, she threw out so many clever, off-color quips that I laughed for days.

Jo's circle of Westport friends looked like they'd stepped fresh out of a J. Crew catalog. Like her, they were unfettered, insouciant, and creative, caring not a whit about what might have killed my husband. With their roll-neck sweaters, wind-tossed hair, and sunny, sandy kids, they seemed free of everything bollixing me right up.

Westport was, of course, the same town I'd fled eight years before, when the bathroom door had locked on Caroline at Robert and Nancy's house and all hell had broken loose. It hadn't occurred to me to live there until seduced by Jo and her photogenic cohort, the idea sweetened by the prospect of Uncle Robert, Aunt Nancy, and their trio of young sons—my children's only cousins—as neighbors.

Connecticut's "gold coast" was hardly our most affordable option, with its lush green fields and sandy beaches. But the public schools were top of the line and the people—well, the people were just who I wanted to be. Elated, Jo sprang into action and in record time found us the perfect turn-of-the-century, walk-to-town, fixer-upper, below-budget saltbox.

That August, we moved.

Dear Baby,

Congratulations on making it through. You did it! You are a trooper and you still sparkle. Love you.

Johnski

Nine

Commuting from Connecticut to my job in Manhattan was not something I'd exactly thought through before moving. Why would I? Jo and her friends didn't commute. Most didn't even work, or worked part-time at home.

But there I was, sixty-seven minutes on Metro North, twice a day, five days a week. I usually caught the 5:18 a.m. train, to hit the gym before work. Dave, who had been downsized shortly after our move, drove me to the train each morning in fuzzy slippers, one hand warmed by a steaming mug.

At the station there were only a handful of women taking the train as early as I, including Marsha, a corporate lawyer and the mother of one of Dan's third-grade friends. Each morning before the sun rose, we stood respectfully apart on the frigid, dark train platform. We eyed each other furtively over our pashmina mufflers, grunting "hello" and juggling our tote bags and newspapers, too tired and cold to talk. All the other people on the platform were men; men in big black overcoats, chatting with other men in a big black overcoats. They bounced up and down, stamping their feet emphatically in the cold.

Once on the train, I looked around at my commuting compadres in their gleaming Italian shoes and cashmere scarves, and mused about what it would be like had John lived. Would I look like those other women in town, tennis-toned and sun-kissed even in winter? Would I be drowsily making coffee in my open-concept kitchen while John went off to work, instead of huddling for warmth on a cracked vinyl seat, pulling my frayed discount overcoat tighter around my thickening middle and wondering if my blouse was buttoned right?

Fortunately, I loved my job. I loved my mostly female bosses and colleagues. I even loved Dave, who was safe, so dramatically different from John. But along with the love, I also resented him. I resented that his lackluster career forced me to be the breadwinner while he was the one raising the kids. *My* kids! At PTA meetings and back-to-school nights, they knew Dave, not me. "Who's she?" I once heard someone ask. "The mother?"

Dave was friendly, relaxed. He had time to make friends in town. I was tired, busy, burdened with secrets. At one school meeting, when I asked a woman how she knew Dave, she collegially tossed her arm around his shoulders and squeezed. "From the dog park," she said. "We're dog people!" I loved our rescue mutt Jenny, but never had a minute to pet her. Who had time to be a dog person? I was a work person. *The* work person.

In other ways, too, Westport was not what I had imagined. With our schedules so different, Jo and I rarely connected. By the following September, Jo and Drew's house was on the market. Drew's production company had gone belly up, they were divorcing, and Jo had relocated herself and her kids to a rental in the next town. Not long after that, she met someone else and moved even farther away.

I never stopped missing Jo after she moved. There wasn't anyone else who, if I told her my husband had died of AIDS, would come back with a joke. There wasn't anyone else in town I could tell that my husband had died of AIDS, period.

As in Hoboken, pristine "small town" Westport made me close up all over again. From the front lines of AIDS, the news was good: miraculous, lifesaving drugs had arrived. But in Connecticut, people still flinched at its mention. One day, Dan came home from a playdate smarting from his friends jeering at an anti-AIDS commercial on TV. "And I couldn't even say anything back," he said ruefully. He was right, he couldn't. I'd taught him well.

I kept my head down, too, and after making a few good friends with whom I formed a book group, I didn't let many other people in. Plus, I wasn't quite sure where I fit in. It certainly wasn't at the beach, I decided, full of women with money and nannies and successful husbands, their glistening legs tucked neatly beneath toned bottoms. They were sleek and effortless; I was messy and tired. They were chattering and gossiping; I was holding my tongue. I reverted to my old Hoboken habit of leaving birthday parties and sleepover pickups early to avoid having to greet people. I mastered the quick slip whenever conversation veered uncomfortably close to questions such as, "Is Dave the father of your children?" or "Who do your kids look like?" All it would take was one slip, one mention to the wrong person.

As I'd settle into my seat on the train every morning, I'd snap open my copy of *The New York Times* with relief. At least no one could discover my secret here. This was my refuge from prying neighbors, hard-charging bosses, demanding children, and mounting concerns about my dying father's cardiopulmonary disease, dying mother's Alzheimer's, and the future welfare of my dependent brother. I lost myself in articles about home design and what was hot on Broadway. Occasionally, though, a headline would scream "AIDS." I'd sink low in my seat, my heart pounding. Could anyone see what I was reading? Dan played football, Caroline swam on the high school team—what if a parent in the seat behind me made the connection? It took a while to settle myself after spotting one of these headlines, to keep my heart from racing. But I still had to read every word, every syllable. It was about me.

In the early years of my commute, these articles were full of death tolls and obituaries, or were focused on gay men wrestling with grief. When articles about survival rates and "cocktails" started to surface—breakthrough treatments that kept people from dying—it was difficult to grasp. I could only equate AIDS with death. There was also the radically changing world of sexuality: a world of Ellen DeGeneres and *Will and Grace*, then *Modern Family* and gay and lesbian wedding announcements. But I wasn't changing in quite the same way, or at quite the same rate. Sometimes I'd sneak—alone, furtively, like a flasher—into movies about closeted homosexuality and AIDS: *Far from Heaven* and *Brokeback Mountain*. I didn't want to be seen. If the film's story included an irreparably wounded, scarred woman, then I *was* that woman. I was that woman, but no one could know.

And yet, as the years passed, John lingered, persistently. Stubbornly. As hard as I tried to shut him out, he continued to haunt my dreams; I thought of him a million times a day. What would *he* think of *Will and Grace*? Were he alive, would he be sitting next to me on the couch watching it, or flipping past it, afraid to be seen liking it? Or would he be watching it, instead, with a boyfriend, laughing uproariously? In school auditoriums, as the lights dimmed and I watched our two adorable kids sing holiday songs or win awards, I'd fight back tears and cry out, soundlessly, "Where are you, John? You're missing this! You're missing so much!"

I wondered all kinds of things about John, like what kind of father he would have been. I considered asking Robert, but how would Robert know what kind of "anything" his brother would have been? He could merely speculate, too. I wanted to be done with John and his secrets, I'd tell my friends. "So get over him, already," they'd respond. *Why can't I do that?* I'd pester myself. *Why can't I be done?*

I knew the answer. John was the man of my dreams, the father of my children, and I couldn't let go of what might have been. I wanted Dan and Caroline to know the man John was before he was sick: the *über*-competent journalist on the rise, the man with whom I fell in love. Supporting this effort was a cadre of John's Brown University friends and *Wall Street Journal* colleagues. We'd meet them for lunch on school breaks, and they'd invite us for weekends at their summer places, when they'd regularly share humorous, admiring anecdotes about him.

And every summer, the four of us joined Robert's family at the old New Hampshire farmhouse where, together with Robert's New England cousins, we picked blueberries, hiked, and barbecued. I'd always sneak away with the kids to visit their father's grave, where they'd stand in shy attention, sneakered feet pressed together, chubby hands offering up tired-looking daisies.

They'd sing songs they learned in school or camp of the "Make new friends, but keep the old" variety. It was peaceful there, in the quiet hush of the country cemetery, far from questions and judgments. Beneath his dignified tombstone, John could become someone I recognized again. I wanted to think of him in this way, to erase any memory of disease and deceit. These visits to his grave provided a flickering moment of fantasy. For a time, I also had John's name called at our synagogue each March, commemorating the anniversary of his death so we could formally, solemnly, and, in the sparsely attended *Shabbat* service, nearly anonymously mourn him.

But by high school, the kids' lives and summers filled up. They pushed back against going to New Hampshire, and to the synagogue, and against any insertion of their phantom, rogue father into their lives. After their award ceremonies and championship games, when I'd tell them how proud he would have been, they'd shrug. "C'mon, Mom. What are you, on drugs? We don't want to talk about him." And really, why would they? This guy, who'd never been there for their skinned knees, swim meets, and proms, was a dirty secret they'd inherited—and that, in their eyes, so had I. Instead, it was always Dave at their concerts and games and award ceremonies. Dave, along with Nancy and Robert, who could usually be counted on to attend, and my father. Flushed with applause, the kids would hug everyone, give Dave a high-five, and then ask, "Pop here?" He always was, beaming as he shuffled slowly up the aisle from his auditorium seat.

He was, that is, until 2004, when, exhausted from caring for my mother, who had died the year before, brokenhearted by her loss, and worried about the welfare of my brother, his lungs, heart, and will to live finally gave out.

After my father's death, I spent months shuttling from Westport to Philadelphia to settle his affairs, sell his house, and help my brother, Bill, move into his own apartment for the first time in his fifty-one years. I handled it all like a skilled juggler, keeping the many balls aloft until finally one slipped from my grasp: I lost my job.

Suddenly, I no longer had to take the 5:18 to the city. I was no longer needed in Philadelphia by my parents or Bill. One of my kids had left for college, the other nearly so. The summer loomed ahead and I had nothing but time.

July fourth that year was blindingly hot and sunny. Dave and I had nothing to do; on holiday weekends, everyone gathered with family, and family was where we ran thin. I suggested we go to the local beach where Dan taught sailing. Since our move to Westport, Dan had spent a good bit of each summer out on the water with Robert, an avid sailor, and his cousins, as well as every August at a rustic boys' camp in the New Hampshire woods to— poetically, for me—sail on Lake Winnipesaukee.

Dan loved to sail. How many times had he asked us to join him on the water, and we'd always found some excuse? Dave liked the beach even less than I did. Whenever I tepidly invited him to go with me, he pulled out one of his "Indiana excuses": "I'm from Indiana—we don't take too well to the sun," or "I'm from Indiana—we don't like taking off our clothes outside." He was kidding, but only by half.

If Dave and I were going to the beach that hot July day, we were going to run the three miles there, I determined. No time like the present to start getting in shape. Nearly one hour later, we heaved and sweated our way up to the dock, where Dan was deep in conversation with a gaggle of red-shirted sailing instructors. When he saw us, he disengaged and made his way over. I became mesmerized by his face, half masked by huge Oakley sunglasses. Dan was a mirror image of his father, who, twenty-two years before, had stood on that very same shore, wearing similarly oversize sunglasses. Ray-Bans, of course.

It was the summer I was pregnant with Caroline; Robert and Nancy had offered us their house while they vacationed. John and I had leapt at the offer, eager to escape our hot Hoboken apartment. While there, John, ever the self-improvement junkie, had decided to learn windsurfing. Queasy and beginning to show, I was more than happy to watch him—devotedly, lovingly—from the dock. During his first and second lessons, John had struggled to balance on the board. He would tip over, get up, then topple again. But by lesson three he was gliding with ease and grace. This man was a marvel, so good at everything he tried.

Now his tall, strong son, Dan, was hustling Dave and me onto a "catamaran"—a piece of cloth stretched between two boards—and making me nervous by gracefully hopping aboard only after we'd disengaged from shore and the water began rhythmically, insistently moving us out. I slipped and slid, one of the flip-flops I'd brought for the voyage landing in the churning waves. Dave—who'd likely wagered we'd end up castaways and would need supplies (I wasn't so sure he was wrong)—struggled to hold on to two bottles of Evian as well as his iPod, his arms and legs akimbo. We all laughed; Dave could make anything funny.

But then we were sailing, Dan masterfully steering us between speedboats, kayaks, and buoys into open water. "Move to the left, guys," he advised calmly. Then: "In a minute I'll need to you to move right. Watch out for that pulley, Dave. You're sitting on it. Not that one, the blue one." Dan was calm, sure, nothing less than a master of his boat, the sea—and us, his insecure elders. Dan, I realized, was like his father.

When Dan entered his senior year of high school that fall, I began to seriously weigh whether it was finally time to reintroduce John into our family's conversation, and into our lives. Things in Westport were going surprisingly well. My long tenure at work had provided enough severance to keep the pressure of a job hunt temporarily at bay. I had time to exercise when and where I wanted, cook nutritious meals, and—for the first time since both kids were tiny—I was home in the afternoon; Dan could finally chuck that latchkey. Dave had snagged a sales job, bringing in money and keeping him cheerfully productive. I was finally becoming engaged in the community, happily vying for every football and track team volunteer opportunity and attending after-school practices, easing my own now slimming behind onto the bleachers with the other moms to dish about the math teacher no one liked, the best farmers' market stand for bread, and, of course...husbands.

Everyone talked about their spouses, even those whom they'd divorced. It was our own sort of sport, dishing about husbands and ex-husbands high up in those stadium stands. And I thought, *Can I? Can I finally join the chorus? Is it time?* Then I'd cast my eyes down on the lush playing field to see my son tossing the pigskin around, laughing and joking, leading the normal life he deserved, and I'd realize, *Not yet.* All it would take was one Susan, one Beth.

None of us deserved that, least of all Dan and Caroline.

One year later, in 2009, Caroline mentioned her father at the seminal moment of her college graduation. There she was, on the campus where her father had once been happy, her diminutive five-foot-three-inch frame engulfed by a massive graduation robe. That fall, she would be going to medical school. She was no longer my little girl, but a wise young woman who'd given herself license to connect with the ghost of her father.

Three years after that, on a verdant campus thirty miles east of Los Angeles, Dan received his college diploma and said, his blue eyes glistening, "Mom, you know who I thought of during the whole ceremony? My father."

At last. It was time. That summer, when both kids were home, I sprung into action, lugging three heavy, taped-up boxes up from the basement. Out came John's pictures and clips and love letters. Out came baby Dan's *Wall Street Journal* birth announcement. Out came the John I'd loved and married before AIDS. Out came everything, and onto the dining room table it went. "Look!" I said. "Here's your father hiking the Rockies! Look, here he is with his old girlfriend in Mill Valley! And look, here's his juicer, and what are these? His gravity boots! Can you believe he had gravity boots?!"

My kids couldn't back away fast enough. "Mom, we don't need to see this now," Caroline said. And they went out for Mexican food.

I sat at the table motionless for hours afterward, wearing John's felt fedora, dented from storage.

A few days later, as I stood looking at the piles on the table, Caroline came up from behind and put her hand on my shoulder. "This stuff doesn't mean anything to us, Mom," she said gently. "You had a relationship with him, but we still have to figure ours out." She was right, I realized. If she and Dan were to someday find a connection to their father, it would be their own, without me. I slowly repacked the boxes, feeling a fresh wave of loneliness.

Soon the kids left, one for another year of medical school, the other for an apartment and job in the city. The tiny Connecticut house became cavernous. With Caroline and Dan gone, Dave and I had little in common. Having lost the sales job, he spent countless hours in his basement office chasing leads for another. I was unemployed again, too, having left another publishing job that required too many hours yet paid too little.

And I was tired. Tired of wrestling with my secret. Tired of spending two full decades alternately longing for John and hating him. Tired of him haunting my dreams. Tired of my mixed-up feelings for the man who replaced him, and who was different from John in so many ways.

I began to write as a way to search for answers. Every morning I made a beeline for my laptop, where I sat hunched over, wearing the same flannel Lanz of Salzburg nightgown day after day, writing about everything I hadn't talked about for nineteen years. The real story about what happened to my marriage, and to John. How angry I was that my life hadn't worked out the way he'd promised. How grateful I still was, every day, that the children and I had been spared. I wrote about how John had burdened me with a disease he'd denied even having, a disease that had foisted me into the darker, more secretive side of male homosexuality— a world now profoundly altered by everything from advances in

AIDS treatment to gay marriage laws, to television shows like *Modern Family* and, astoundingly, *Girls Who Like Boys Who Like Boys*. A world to which I desperately needed to catch up.

One Saturday, Dan came by for a visit and found me in my usual position, hunched over my computer in an unwashed nightgown. "Mom," he said gently, "get out of here. Get out of here, already."

So I did. I told Dave I needed some time, and set off for my own tiny rental apartment in Manhattan. My son was right. It was time to set myself free.

"Love to love you, baby."
John
P.S. Your transition will be transcendent, okay?

Ten

By moving to my own apartment in the city, I wasn't just breaking away from Dave and shedding my suburban existence and rancid Lanz of Salzburg nightie. I was, as my *AARP* magazine incessantly hounded me, "reinventing!"

I landed a flex-time job that paid a decent salary while providing time to try some new "me"s on for size and enrolled in a graduate-level linguistics class at a university downtown. I took tap dance classes at a Y uptown. I trained for the New York City Marathon in the park, three blocks away. I joined a synagogue that promised access to a diverse, socially active community. I thought about dating. I hadn't just left Dave; in a sense, he'd left me, too. Emphatically opposed to living in Manhattan again, he was determined to stay in Westport. I was ambivalent about living without him in the city, but not one whit ambivalent about going there to start my next chapter. Dave could stay in the house if he could afford it. I needed to see what—and, very possibly, who—was out there waiting for me.

I could barely catch my breath as I flitted from one activity to another. Ironically, I became a lesson junkie like John, with his jazz piano, windsurfing, and seductive swim lessons. John, who, if I could succeed in reinventing myself into a fabulous new me, I could finally leave behind.

One night soon after my move to the city, racked by my usual insomnia, I grabbed the TV remote and clicked onto a film called *We Were Here*. "What's this?" I mused, half conscious, as image after image of muscular men flashed across the screen: men hugging and dancing, men marching and yelling, men skeletal and dying. "Oh no, not again," I heard myself say, yanking the sheets over my face and then lowering a corner to continue watching. It was a documentary about the early years of the AIDS epidemic in San Francisco. I watched the whole thing, then clicked over to Nick at Nite, where I knew reruns of *The Nanny* could be depended on for laughs until five-thirty, when I would head out to the park for my four-mile training run.

But when I got out to the park that morning, I couldn't budge more than a few feet on my usual route. I'd take some steps, then stop cold. Run, stop. A few more steps, stop. I felt like lead. What was happening?

Disgusted with myself, I headed to the neighborhood Starbucks for my usual venti, and then home. When I arrived, I forgot about work, tap class, and a looming take-home linguistics quiz, and sat at my new Pottery Barn table, motionless. Images from the film ran through my head. Those beautiful men, sick and dying. Eloquent, grief-stricken survivors, testifying how their lives had changed forever. These men had borne witness to the AIDS-riddled 1980s and '90s. They had been robbed of the young, promising men of their dreams. Well, so had I.

I had never taken my place in their world, but, I saw with crystalline clarity, I needed to now. Otherwise, as in the park that morning, I would never be able to move forward. John's disease was a secret I no longer wanted to keep. I had to square up with it, own it, take my rightful place as its witness. My tap shoes lay dusty on the floor as I began to channel every moment once earmarked for "reinvention" into the singular pursuit of connecting with AIDS, searching for one single kernel of meaning in it. For me.

The time felt right. It was the twenty-fifth anniversary of AIDS and New York was awash in museum exhibits, movies, and plays, the hottest ticket being the twenty-fifth anniversary Broadway production of Larry Kramer's play *The Normal Heart*, profiling the early days of HIV in New York City. Back in 1985, when the play had first been produced, it had barely appeared on my radar. Why would it? I was engaged to be married, busy finding a wedding venue. This time around, I got a third-row center seat, then sat and cried. Many around me sobbed audibly. When the lights came up, I looked around and saw almost all men, many tenderly holding hands. Nothing new there—except me. I was there, and accountable, instead of sneaking out before the lights came up. This was progress.

Progress, that is, except that I was lonelier than ever, sitting among the sea of men that night. I was missing my own. I missed Dave. This mission to connect with my past was hard enough without Dave's solid, dependable form nearby. Happily, Dave joined me for my next foray, a well-publicized exhibit at the New-York Historical Society called "AIDS in New York: The First Five Years." We arrived early, expecting to find a line spilling out the door. Instead, we practically had the place to ourselves. As we toured the museum's majestic halls, the sound of my heels echoed on the marble floors. The place was a tomb.

Where was everybody?

I began reading magazines like *POZ*, for HIV-positive people, and *OUT*, a magazine for gays and lesbians. I read AIDS-related fiction by Paul Monette and Edmund White. I watched Tony Kushner's brilliant *Angels in America*, in which Mary-Louise Parker plays Harper Pitt, the denial-laden wife of a still-closeted husband. In other words: me. I'd never seen myself in an AIDS-related movie or play before.

When I read a glowing review in *The New York Times* of an Oscar-nominated documentary called *How to Survive a Plague* that was playing in Greenwich Village—in this case, a neighborhood of historic importance—I rushed for tickets and this time enlisted my son, who lived near the theater, to join me, albeit reluctantly. I'd given the film a massive buildup, hoping it would shed light for both of us on the magnitude of the epidemic that had killed his father, but was mortified to find only a handful of people there. At a movie about AIDS in Greenwich Village? Was everybody brunching?

Empty museums, empty movie theaters. It was like throwing a party and having no one come. Was I seeking closure on something that was, in fact, closed for business? I felt a tad red-faced, foolhardy, chasing some affiliation with a disease my husband, its victim, hadn't even copped to.

I put my mission on ice and switched to training for the New York City Marathon. When his work schedule permitted, Dan joined me on my longer runs. One beautiful day in May, while running through Central Park, he and I were waylaid by a stream of foot soldiers carrying banners with slogans like "Silence = Death" and "We miss you, Ricardo." "It's the AIDS Walk," I whispered. The AIDS Walk. Why had I never done it? Why, of course, I wouldn't have done it—wouldn't have wanted to be seen doing it. But here they were, all these people—young, old, all races and cultures—walking for AIDS. A cluster of women passed wearing t-shirts that read "AIDS Widows."

"That's your group, Mom," Dan said.

I felt a chill. My *group*? I had no group when it came to AIDS, did I? I looked at the women holding the cards. They had been widowed by AIDS, too, but they weren't skulking in the shadows. I suddenly wanted to fall in step and say, "Me, too!" Instead, I grabbed Dan's forearm. "Let's do this next year," I said. "Can we?" And like the good son he is, he said yes.

Peace. Love you.
John

Eleven

One year later, Dan and I formed our own AIDS Walk group of two. To raise money in pledges "in memory of John Andrew," I decided to post the news of our participation—and thus of John's having died of AIDS—on Facebook. This would mean, for the first time, outing him—outing us, actually—to my six hundred friends, several of whom were also Dan's and Caroline's. Everyone would know what killed "Andrew," and I would be telling them. It was John's prophecy, come true. Should I do it?

Too often I could be found wasting time on Facebook. It was an addiction, to feast off the happenings of other people's lives. I posted once in a while myself, though I was vigilant about doing so zealously, wary of stirring up "fear of missing out" (or "FOMO," as my kids say) in my friends. I didn't want them to feel as I did: jealous when others posted wedding photos captioned "blessed for twenty-five years." I had celebrated my own beautiful wedding twenty-five years ago, too, but had been hiding it ever since. And now I was thinking of posting—what?—on my profile page, for all to see?

I consulted with Dan. Was it okay with him if I broke the truth about his father's illness on Facebook? "Of course, Mom," he answered, without hesitation. Caroline gracefully stepped aside to allow me do it, but her discomfort was apparent. Was she right?

I hesitated, afraid to be "all in." Telling the truth was hard; it could create stress and divisiveness in families. But keeping secrets could also create divisiveness. I knew, because my father's family harbored a big one.

Nearly a century ago, on a snowy night in Asbury Park, New Jersey, my father's father, Albert Kneip, had driven his family's bakery delivery truck into an oncoming train. My dad was four at the time, his little sister, Lillian, two. In a situation eerily similar to that of my own children, they were never to know their own father.

No one seemed to talk about my grandfather after his death—or at least, not to my father. My dad had something to say about everyone, but about his father, he was empty. Everything I know is from this tattered newspaper clipping, which I found in a crumbling box of memorabilia after my father died:

Lets One Train Pass, Is Fatally Hurt by Another
Albert Kneip, Baker, Dies in Hospital After Crash on Munroe Avenue Crossing—Flagman Reported on Duty

Apparently failing to heed the warning of the crossing flagman, Albert Kneip, 34, of 904 Pine Street, associated with his father, William Kneip, in the bakery business at 1200 Munroe Avenue, drove on to death in the path of an onrushing Pennsylvania train at the Munroe Avenue crossing last evening.

The article continues: "Kneip, it is believed, had waited for the northbound train, leaving the Asbury Park Station at 7 o'clock to pass the crossing and then, believing the way was clear had started his car, a Ford delivery, over the tracks. The flagman had then displayed his red lantern and shouted to Kneip as the latter started his car across the tracks. If Kneip saw the warning of the flagman or heard his shouts," the article reports, "he apparently became obsessed with the idea that he could beat the train out."

What kind of man was my grandfather to ignore the flagman's frantic warning? Was he a daredevil, believing he could beat it? Was he exhausted after a long day of delivering bread? Was he inebriated? Was he despondent? Did he want to die?

Again, my father had no opinions or answers concerning his father, provoking me to surmise that his mother, my grandmother, who died when I was eight, hadn't told her son much at all about him, deciding to let his story follow him to the grave.

The accident that killed my grandfather also killed my grandmother's connection with his family. After that tragic, snowy night in 1924, the German-Jewish Kneips strongly urged my bereft, near penniless young grandmother to return to her Polish-Jewish clan, and she whisked her children back to their bosom in Virginia. The relationship eventually dissolved into occasional Jewish New Year greetings, gifts of fresh rolls and other foodstuffs. One lovely cousin stayed in touch, but he didn't—or couldn't—talk about my grandfather, either.

Then: a break! Another cousin visited a relative in Israel (who knew we had relatives in Israel?) who asked, "Where are all the Kneips?" The question prompted him to hunt around for me, and to organize a family reunion of sorts back in Asbury Park, home of the infamous bakery. Among our group were three frail first cousins of my father's, approaching ninety. When I asked one if she knew anything about my grandfather, her uncle, she said, "Well, the suicide theory is pure bunk." "Uncle Alley," she went on to say, had rushed across the tracks that night to pick up medicine for one of his children. The flagman had not warned my grandfather about the train, as the newspaper reported, but had actually fallen asleep. Finally, she proclaimed that the railroad's insurance company forced the newspaper to report the story otherwise, to dodge liability and pay my grandmother the minimum amount of insurance.

Also attending the reunion was our Israeli cousin, Dorit, who had recently discovered a family secret of her own, having come upon letters in an old trunk from her grandparents, about whom her own parents had never spoken. The letters revealed that her grandparents, like many Jews in Antwerp, Belgium, in the early 1940s, had committed suicide before the Nazis could transport them to the camps. Dorit had written a book largely composed of these letters, to honor her grandparents, validate their existence, and make them part of the world again.

Family secrets camouflage situations people can't talk about: suicide, the Holocaust, mental illness, and, of course, AIDS. I didn't want John shrouded similarly. I, too, wanted to validate his life, to make him part of the world again. I wanted truth to be connected to how he died. I wanted truth reinstated in mine.

My Facebook page glowed before me on the screen. I shut my eyes and pressed post.

Seconds later, pledges began pouring in—from friends of John's from Brown that I hadn't heard from since he died, from his colleagues at the *Journal*, from Robert and Nancy and his relatives in New Hampshire, from my own colleagues, from Hoboken neighbors, parents from the Manhattan New School, parents of Dan's and Caroline's college friends, and from several Westport neighbors. Comments such as "In memory of John Andrew, who left us too soon," "We miss you, John," and, "In memory of John Andrew, and in honor of Maggie, Caroline, and Dan" crowded the donation page. When all was said and done, I handed over a sizeable amount to the Gay Men's Health Crisis to benefit people and families afflicted by AIDS who did not get the kind of support I received from family and *The Wall Street Journal*.

On the day of the event, Dan and I stood in a rain-drenched Central Park watching the opening ceremony, shivering among a grieving crowd of not just graying gay men but young people, too, and women—everyone hailing from different cultures and neighborhoods. An actress climbed onto the bandbox and began singing "For Good," from the hit Broadway musical *Wicked*. I'd always found the song a bit cheesy, but as she sang, I found myself sobbing.

"*Who can say if I've been changed for the better, because I knew you,*" she sang, "*because I knew you, I have been changed for good.*"

Standing amid this sea of bedraggled foot soldiers, with my tall, strong son holding his umbrella over me to protect me from the rain, I was suddenly overcome with emotion. Never much of a crier, I was heaving, gasping for breath. For a moment, it was difficult to distinguish my tears from the rain. I felt—for the first time in...how long?—how much I had once loved John.

And how, through the fine children he'd left behind, he had—yes—changed me for good. The wonderful young man by my side, his beautiful, gifted sister—both so like John in their expressions, mannerisms, and, most of all, sharp wit and shining intellects. John may have died from AIDS, leaving me with his terrible secret. But he had also left me with the best of himself: our children.

I couldn't go on hating John, or I'd never let go.

One year later, I joined the AIDS Walk again, this time walking for a women's AIDS organization and raising twice what I had raised the year before. As I walked alongside them, hundreds of them, I heard stories of great courage. Some had survived marriages decimated by AIDS but had been mercifully uninfected, like me. Some had been infected but, saved by lifesaving drugs, were walking strong. And some, despite the new drugs, were nursing severely ill family members, and burying them. Even in this brave new world, not everyone comes forward to get tested and medicated. Condemnation of homosexuality keeps people in the closet, and in denial. People are still dying.

Listening to these women, hearing this brave, new, and decidedly female voice of AIDS, I, too, began talking. I talked to the two women who led our HIV-negative wives' support group in the early 1990s. I talked to people who asked about my past and finally answered them honestly. A surprising number responded that they, too, had lost loved ones to AIDS, especially brothers, whom they'd rarely mentioned until talking with me. I became a confidante for people who'd been silenced, had silenced themselves, or both. Like me.

I talked and talked. When I saw the movie *Dallas Buyers Club*, rather than sneaking out early as I had so many times before, I wrote about how that and so many other movies addressing the AIDS crisis left women victims on the cutting room floor. When my writing was turned into a published article entitled, "My Invisible Life as an AIDS Widow," I was contacted by other women who had also lost husbands to the disease. *Where have you been all my life?* I wondered. Hiding out, most likely.

I not only felt like talking, I felt like singing. How long had it been? Nearly thirty years, ever since crooning with Chris while cleaning up the greasy crabhouse at the end of our shifts. I learned of an adult education course at the Y called "Intro to Cabaret" and signed up.

Our class consisted of a handful of therapists, a human resources executive, a patent attorney, a TV newscaster—Magee Hickey, who was also a local celebrity—and me. We were to select, rehearse, and (once our knees stopped shaking) knock 'em dead with three songs in a seedy Manhattan nightclub, for one night only. Clad in boas, sequins, and red velour, my classmates' song lists included tunes like "Happy Days Are Here Again!" and "I Love a Parade." Mine ran more along the lines of the Who's doleful "The Song Is Over," and "Behind Blue Eyes." I wore black.

One day, Magee, whose own peppy act boasted a cartwheel, cornered me. "What's up?" she asked. "Why are your songs so sad?"

"Yeah, I guess my songs are a bummer," I said. "I'm in the process of working through something...the death of my husband."

"Oh, I'm so sorry. When did he die?" she asked.

My face went slightly red. "A long time ago," I said. "Twenty-two years, to be precise." Magee looked perplexed. "I wasn't really able to talk about it before," I said. "He had AIDS."

"Oh," she said. "Oh."

Anticipating the next question and steeled with my new-found resolve to talk, I determined to head it off at the pass. "I don't have it," I said. "I'm well. And so are our kids." I mentioned that my husband, John Andrew, like her, was a journalist. Did she by any chance know him?

"I went to college with a John Andrew," she said. "Did he go to Brown?"

I nodded, my eyes widening.

"I remember him," Magee replied. "He was a cool guy. He worked on the newspaper and had bright red hair. I used to always see him running across the green. I had no idea he died." She touched my hand. "I was first motivated to sing, myself, two years ago, when my mother died. I couldn't manage to croak out anything but a dirge back then—but it helped. How old are your kids now?"

I told her they were both college graduates, and that neither had had the chance to know their father, who'd died before Dan was even a year old.

"That's too bad," she said. Then she lit up, including her sequins. "Do you know Michael Blumstein?" she asked. "He's a friend of mine, and was a good friend of John's at Brown. They worked together on the paper. I'm going to put you two together."

I actually did know Mike. Back in the day, as they say, John and I had dinner with him and his then fiancée. We had even attended their wedding.

Within days, Mike and I found ourselves perched on stools in a Times Square Starbucks, talking about John. In fact, Mike didn't just talk about John, he crowed about him. He also offered to talk to the kids about their father. We would meet again, we decided, to arrange it.

But we didn't have to. Some months later, a beautiful email arrived for me to forward to the kids, in which Mike described how special—"magical, really"—John was. "Many of us were genuinely blessed to know John," he wrote, "and it would truly sadden us if you didn't have the fullest possible picture of him in your head and heart." Mike went on to describe their father as having "coolness with zero effort," as "ironic but not cynical, witty but not biting," and as having "distinct intellect and creativity." He even attached some of John's articles from their time together at Brown's *Daily Herald*.

"Please know that nearly twenty-three years after your dad was mysteriously grabbed from us," he wrote, "we remember him clearly and miss him dearly. We all meet many, many people in our lives. We meet so few who touch others with true deftness and warmth."

Caroline, Dan, and I all found ourselves similarly moved by Mike's email. "Not many people who knew my father are willing to talk (or write) about him like you did," Dan responded, "and I'm grateful to you for helping to fill some big holes."

"As my mother may have told you," wrote Caroline, "it's been challenging to learn about who my father was, and your letter helps put the pieces together a little bit more."

It was openness that had let this happen, I realized. It was finding my voice. It was telling the truth. How critical it was to bring John back into the conversation.

As I spoke more and more freely about him—and us—an old friend remarked on what a great couple John and I had been.

What if, I wondered, AIDS hadn't been our game changer, our ultimate demise? What if, instead, John had eventually "come out" as gay, or bisexual, in our more tolerant world? Would we have remained together, raising our kids, celebrating our anniversaries, planning our retirement, with our lifestyle and marriage adapting accordingly? It's a nice thought. But that wasn't our reality. His illness, and death, were our reality. They were our game changer—our *ultimate* game changer. As they were for so many other couples ravaged by AIDS.

John was a young, flaming-haired magic man with a blazingly hot future. He loved me and he loved his children, whom he expected to help bring up and to know. He was also a man with a past, a man with conflicted feelings and secret yearnings.

The realities of John's disease kept the end of our marriage from being a beautiful, redemptive one. There were no tear-stained *mea culpa*s, the kind people expect in a tragic love story. The words were left unsaid, the questions never answered. The disease outed a part of John he kept deeply secret, of which he was ashamed. This secrecy and shame swallowed up his legacy, consumed his memory. They robbed us of our right to mourn him.

In telling the truth, I'm now taking that back.

If I could talk to John now, I would tell him how I wished he could have been honest about who he was, but that I understand why he wasn't, given the shame of those years. I would tell him that today the cover story of a major national newspaper was "Bisexual Male Seeking Like-Minded Friends…and Legitimacy: How a New Breed of Activists Is Using Science to Prove There's Something Real Between Straight and Gay." And how a few weeks later, another headline read, "The End of Gaydar."

I would tell him that for the longest time, the most painful moment of my life was when he accused me of giving him AIDS. For years, I searched for an explanation as to why he did this, consulting some of the best psychiatrists and doctors around. They could only point to something called "disinhibition," an impulsive disregard for social conventions that can be caused by brain lesions. In the spirit of letting go, I'll allow for it. It's time.

I would tell him, of course, about the wonderful kids he left behind, whom it was my—and Dave's—privilege to raise.

I'd tell him that today, I am a woman who no longer requires streamlining or silencing—who no longer needs a man to be her editor. As it turned out, "losing the best husband a girl could want" taught this girl that she could do the work herself.

I would also tell John that I know, now, he was just a mortal. A mere mortal. A human being, with a touch more magic than most.

All of these things are true. To hide any part of this truth, from my friends, my family, my kids, or myself, diminishes what I've been through. The good, the bad, and even the ugly—they're all part of life's narrative, if we are brave enough to own them. The notes I sing may be more dissonant than those of the exuberant "Graceland" played on my wedding day, but they make me who I am. All of our stories, our songs, make us who we are.

Today, Caroline is a busy medical resident in a big city hospital, where she sees and treats the ravages of AIDS firsthand. While still a first-year medical student, she wrote me a memorable email: "Mom, I am learning all about HIV and it's so strange," she wrote. "Each week we discuss a case and today it was about an AIDS patient. It's just amazing how people can live with

AIDS now. It's also made me realize how lucky we all are, and how lucky it is that you got pregnant easily! It's just so weird to be learning about viral count and all that and then have to think about it in the context of my own father and how we could all be sick right now."

Caroline, Dan, and I have, at last, begun to talk about John and his death. I'm beyond grateful that we can. We've discussed the anger we sometimes feel—not at John for dying, but at him for dying of a disease we couldn't talk about, making life so much harder to navigate and rendering him a non-memory. The three of us have also discussed how lucky we feel not to be sick, not to be plying ourselves with pills to keep from dying. Dan summed it up best when he recently said, "It's not something I think about every day. But I'll obviously never not think about it."

Dan lives in Santa Monica, California, about three blocks from where his father lived at his age while a young reporter at *The Wall Street Journal*'s Los Angeles bureau. On a visit there recently, we strolled over to John's faceless, mid-century condominium, where I took Dan's picture, and where it occurred to me that one day, like John, I won't be here, either.

What will Caroline and Dan then say about us—about their father—when we're both gone? I'm bequeathing them the boxes (once they live in places big enough to store them). John, their father, is now theirs. Someday they might even want to show him to their kids, and if they do I hope it's without strategic edits or shame. Now that they've grown up in this brave new world, I hope they feel ready to, like me, shake off the fear of stigma when it comes to mentioning their father. And I hope they can get to know the best of him. Friends like Mike Blumstein have certainly given them a good start. Both shared with me that on a recent road trip to California, they read John's personal letters aloud to each other. There's likely no better way to become acquainted with the essence of their father, John Andrew, an uncommonly smart, funny writer—and man. I could not have been more delighted.

I recently moved back to Connecticut, where the living is easy—mainly because I am. I no longer swim against the current of worry and fear. Instead, I swim at the beach whenever I can and enjoy it. I've gotten to know more people in town because I no longer loathe the dreaded questions. I savor telling the truth. After all this time, the truth feels like a privilege. A gift.

As it turned out, Dave couldn't live without me, and I couldn't live without him, either. This sweet, funny man who helped me raise such fine children, caringly nurse and bury my parents, guide my brother into independent living, and who keeps me laughing day after day, was another part of my story—one that I didn't want to end. Dave has finally turned his back on sales and, as we should have foreseen years ago, found his calling with kids, reading aloud to students in local schools (using a different voice for each character, of course). This still leaves me as the official breadwinner, but as long as Dave makes me laugh, I'm okay with that. Recently he suggested I entitle this book *Shit Out of Luck*, and he may not be wrong. Then he suggested he write his own book and call it *How to Be Boring*.

A man who tells it like it is? Music to my ears.

Often, Dave and I are asked if we're ever going to get married. And though the institution of marriage is a sacred and beautiful one, for me, the moment seems to have passed. Dave and I are good the way we are, honest and committed. Which, when you come down to it, is pretty close to how a marriage should be. We are also pretty much all each other has. Dave has four sisters, but we rarely see three of them. On my side, we enjoy a dependable, convivial relationship with Robert and Nancy, as well as a smattering of cousins. We enjoy the occasional weekend with my brother, Bill. And of course, there are "the kids," to whom, like so many parents, we sometimes cling for dear life. But in the dark, in trouble, in times of need, it's me and Dave. We have each other.

As we're getting on in years, our metabolisms more sluggish than ever, I've taken to exercising even earlier in the morning, leaving Dave snoring in bed. When I pat his mid-section and encourage him to join, he says, "Love handles? Really? I think I look good." We could all use a little more of what Dave's got, that satisfaction with what is. Once he saves enough money to buy a new Martin guitar, well, for him things will be just about perfect.

As for me, I am still seeking balance in ballet class, piano lessons, and singing—even an occasionally upbeat tune in a club act I perform around Manhattan, accompanied by an old Hoboken friend, who happens to be a world-class pianist, and his A-list musician friends, each and every one a star. Just standing on the same stage, I can feel their luminescence.

But it's not about stars anymore, really. Sorry, Mom. It's not about that at all, I've found. Nor is it about perfection, the kind I once craved. It's about loving, losing, and letting go. It's about courage. It's about speaking the truth.

Today, when people ask how my husband died, I just go ahead and tell them. And I think, *Perfect.*

Afterword

BY DR. DALE ATKINS

As a psychologist, media mental health commentator, and edu-
cator, I treat women on a daily, if not hourly, basis with countless
issues that set their lives off balance.

Because there are just so many hours in a day, and far too
many people to help when they need it most, I wrote a book,
Sanity Savers: Tips for Women to Live a Balanced Life, presenting
365 issues—one for each day of the year—brought regularly
to me by women patients and viewers alike, along with their
possible solutions. The issues range from how to relate to your
mother-in-law to how to manage an eating disorder to how to
reveal your child is gay, each accompanied by varying degrees of
the same challenges: how to come to terms with the issue, how
to communicate it, and how to face it honestly, without denial.

But even with 365 issues addressed in my book, it wasn't until
I met Maggie Kneip that I realized I'd left out a whopper: AIDS.

Like thousands of others who lived during that horrific disease's peak, I'd been deeply touched by its tragedy. Professionally,

it reached me through my treatment of gay male patients and of women dealing with the loss of uncles, brothers, and sons. I knew of very few husbands dying of AIDS, though, in the context of treatment. Nor was this particular issue part of the high-profile national AIDS conversation. It was a topic barely whispered.

Talk about something that could set a woman's life reeling. Talk about an unwieldy secret—a massive communications problem. Then picture Maggie. The fact that her husband was dying of AIDS, a largely male homosexual, communicable, fatal disease, put her in another league. No, not a league. With this issue, she was on her own. Isolated.

Maggie and I met at a dinner party one snowy February night in 2001, and instantly warmed to each other. Aware of my profession, and as a new resident in town and the mother of two preteen children, she confided in me about the challenges she faced in keeping the cause of their father's death a secret. Innocent questions from the Welcome Wagon, including "What does your husband do?" and "Is this your kids' dad?" prompted the need to obfuscate and lie. Every PTA meeting and Little League game was a minefield.

But it wasn't long before I saw that Maggie was adept at handling her secret, and over the next nearly two decades, I observed her negotiate it deftly, while raising two strong, secure, successful children and handling a full-time job. When her life issues became even more complicated, as they inevitably do, involving elder dementia, sibling disability, and job loss, she stayed strong, even training for a marathon, understanding the importance of caring for herself, so she could better care for others.

How did she do this?

Maggie would be the first person to tell you that, although she often felt very much alone, she didn't do it alone. Quite the opposite. She took on a loyal, caring partner and de facto stepfather for her children. She sought professional help, medically and psychologically. She connected, frequently and honestly, with her children's educators. She communicated as openly as possible with her children, as well as with her family and her late husband's family. She learned whom to trust, then pulled these people into a close-knit group, of which, I'm pleased and honored to say, I am one.

Best of all, she never lost her sense of humor.

I learned something, watching her. Or rather, watching her reconfirmed something for me. Maggie's near-catastrophic encounter, in her youth, with her husband's horrific, unspeakable illness and death provided her with a boot camp for life. It gave her basic training in maintaining her sanity through any issue life could throw her way, including the loss of her mother to another closeted disease, Alzheimer's, and her brother's long-denied disability—issues many of us face in our lives and families.

This wonderful book, *Now Everyone Will Know*, is really just a chapter in a life that could be any of ours. At some point, we must break free from secrets that cripple us—stop us in our tracks—to maintain sanity. We must reconsider our lives to move on. How Maggie did this, as depicted in her book, is a model for us all.

For those faced with the difficult challenge of managing secrets in their lives, I want to take this opportunity to recommend the helpful work of authors who can guide you toward a more mindful approach: Tara Brach, Brene Brown, Pema Chödrön, Thich Nhat Hanh, Jon Kabat-Zinn, Daniel Siegel, and Jack Kornfield. Following this afterword, you can also find reader's guide questions that probe the challenging issue of managing personal and family secrets.

Reading *Now Everyone Will Know* has reminded me that as the world turns and changes, so do our problems and their solutions. One thing, however, remains the same: by being truthful with ourselves—and when the time is right—we can, as did Maggie, release a secret and achieve, beyond a sense of balance, a redemptive and restorative state of grace.

With the right mix of hope, courage, honesty, and humor, this lovely state of being is within all of our grasps.

DR. DALE ATKINS

September 2015
New York City
www.drdaleatkins.com

Reading Group Guide

- In Maggie's youth, she is cautioned by her father against being too fat or funny. Considering the confident swagger and commercial success of such young female performers today as Lena Dunham and Amy Schumer, is it a more acceptable time for women to relax their standards on behavior and body type? Has society relaxed its standards to accommodate? If so, how? How do men feel about women who act and look in ways that are outside the "norm"?

- Do you think Maggie should have probed more into John's background before she married him? When entering a relationship, how extensively should one investigate a potential partner's history? Given that Maggie and John's encounter was before smartphones, how has today's technology altered this prospect? Are there hazards of online dating? What are they? And finally, how well do any of us know our significant others? Is complete transparency always the goal?

- What do you think of John? Should he have been honest with Maggie about having slept with men when she asked? As someone who had committed his professional life to exposing the truth about others, why do you think he steadfastly covered up the truth about himself? Do you empathize with him for not being honest about it at the time?

- Why do you think John falsely accused Maggie in the hospital? Why do you think he didn't communicate with her during his illness, when he appeared to be able to do so with others?

- Do you feel Maggie's anger at John during his illness was warranted? Was her decision to cease living with and caring for him full-time, during the nine months he lived after his diagnosis, warranted?

- Was Maggie's feeling of isolation due to the disease that killed her husband legitimate? Could she have done a better job of finding women like her? Do you know—or have you known—any women or mothers affected by AIDS through marriage? If so, how did they handle the situation?

- What do you consider the single biggest challenge Maggie faced during her husband's illness?

- Do you think Maggie was right in telling her children the truth of how their father died when they entered school at age five? How honest should we be, or can we be, with our children about situations in our lives that may affect them?

- After John's death, Maggie chose a partner, Dave, with the welfare of her children in mind. What are the challenges a parent faces in bringing a stepparent into the family?

- In her relationship, Maggie is uncomfortable about being the primary breadwinner while Dave serves as "Mr. Mom." Raised by a mother who worked, Maggie takes pride in being a working mother, yet also feels embittered about having to support the man in her life—a feeling reinforced during her early morning commute, where she is surrounded by men while the wives stay home. What do you think of this feeling? Is it more applicable to another time? What factors in Maggie's life may have exacerbated this feeling?

- While still a young mother, Maggie is expected to care for John. Eventually, on top of her job, she becomes responsible for caring for her elderly parents, as well as her older brother. Discuss the expectations of society for women today, which often include financially supporting and caring for family members of separate generations. Should more help be provided for working women by their employers or by government? Is this happening already?

- Maggie was wary of the stigma of AIDS until her children graduated from high school, some fifteen years after John died. By then, major medical strides had been made in treating and managing the disease, as well as in society's acceptance of it. Was Maggie's prolonged wariness of this stigma warranted?

- What do you feel had the greatest impact in allowing Maggie to release her anger and reconsider John and how he died? Was it her children's observations at their respective college graduations? Her awakening to the changing world around her? The break she took from Dave and her suburban life to focus on herself? When faced with the need for change in one's life, if one is unable to afford the time and expense to break away, how else might it be achieved?

- Attitudes toward homosexuality, bisexuality, and transgender lifestyles are changing in many parts of the world. Could you accept your children embracing a transgender lifestyle? How best can we communicate that situation to others?

- Increasingly, celebrities are publicly sharing their sexuality and lifestyle choices. How do you feel about this? How does it affect us—and our children?

- Maggie is compelled to reveal the truth about how John died, in part because she does not want to perpetuate a history of family secrets. Is her concern warranted? How might we be affected by secrets kept in families? Are there family secrets that might be legitimate to keep? What do we do when there's a family secret we want to reveal, but others in the family disagree?

- Maggie believes in being honest, and moreover, that there is a "right time" to be so. Do you agree? When should we keep a secret, and when is the right time to share it?

- Maggie doesn't believe she'll marry again. Do you think this is a result of the traumatic result of her marriage to John? How important is it for her to be married to Dave, now that the children are grown? In a time of newfound marriage equality, has the importance of marriage intensified in people's eyes?

Acknowledgments

This book would not have been possible without the support of so many trusted, smart, and generous friends and colleagues.

First, my deepest thanks go to the family members who unceasingly advocated, protected, and defended, without flinching, during the course of John's illness and in its aftermath: the late Carolyn and Arthur Kneip, Nancy Yates, and Robert Andrew. Thanks also to Nancy and Robert for the love and care they provide my children to this day.

Thank you to those who exquisitely supported me by running by my side in those harrowing early days, including my beloved Y jogging posse of Bonnie Anthony, the Reverend Lucia Ballantine, Cathy Cuthell, the late, lovely Lyn Witheford, Denise Yost, and our locker room pal Jane Musky. Thanks also to Harry Allen, Travis Anderson, David Anthony, Tim Athan, Mary Ellen Atkinson, Patrick Atkinson, Elizabeth Avedon, Mark Basile, Leon Berton, Brett Blau, the late Gabe Carucci, Ray Carucci, Candice Chaplin, Tom Cirolia, John Colianni, David Cuthell, Bernadette

Dempsey, Elvira Diaz, Dan German, Tony Goldwyn, Jane Hammerslough and Ezra Palmer, Harry Harkin, Paula Harkin, Carol Harmon and Ieuan Mahony, the Reverend Margaret Hodgkins and Robinson Hodgkins, Kelley Holland, Sarah Holmes, the late Eugene Kahn, Michael Kahn, the late Tom King, Christina Klotz, Rachel Atkinson Marrin, Debra Mayer, Ruth Mayer, Judy Newman and Jeff MacGregor, Mary Mower Mitchell, Christine O'Day, Michelle Atkinson Pachos, Scot J. Paltrow, Jessalyn Peters, Tim Peters, Noel Rubinton, Celia Ruiz, Jessica Sanders, Steven Schnepp, Tom Tisch, and Karl Woitach.

Thanks to my *Wall Street Journal* dream team, so at the ready—and so incredibly kind—including Byron Calame, Alix Freedman, Joanne Lipman, Norman Pearlstine, Johnnie Roberts, Paul Steiger, and the paper's entire Media and Marketing section staff of those years.

I am grateful to my incomparable medical dream team, including Drs. Jeffrey Gumprecht, Sharon Lewin, Eric Neibart, Sylvia Olarte, and Laura Popper.

The wonderful educators at the Manhattan New School, P.S. 290, impacted us so positively during the critical years of 1993 to 1998. Thank you to Joan Backer, Judy Davis, Principal Shelley Harwayne, Layne Hudes, Eve Mutchnik, Karen Ruzzo, and Joanne Hindley Salch.

For their support of everything I do, including this book, my deepest gratitude goes out to Laura Landro and Dr. Dale Atkins, and their husbands, Richard Salomon and Robert Rosen, respectively.

This book simply wouldn't exist without the loyal support of my cherished publishing colleague and dear friend Sean Cassidy.

It also might not have happened without the "never say die" mentality instilled in me on bitterly cold winter mornings by personal trainer extraordinaire Thomas Baldwin III, a worldly-wise young man if ever there was one.

Michael Blumstein, you know how I feel about you. John was lucky to know you, and we are, too.

Others who have played critical roles in the writing of this book, whom I profoundly thank, include Amelia Atlas, Carol Isaacson Barash, Ellie Berger, Collette Black, Linda Carlson, Alan Cohen, Claire Cohen, Dorit Cohen, Hettie Cohen, Caren Copening, Julie Curtis, Paula Derrow, Rebecca Distler, Deloris Dockrey, Trudy Elins, Michal Eshed, Andrea Fine, Jessica Foroutan, Alix Freedman, Kelli Gail, Ken Geist, Bill and Mitzi Gilman, Jon Gilman, John Glassie, Judy Goldberg, Rachel Goldberg, Katori Hall, the late Sarah Herz, Magee Hickey, Janet and Leonard Horowitz, Peggy Intrator, Carolyn Jackson, Melissa Kirsch, Julia Klein, Loni Klein, Jerry Kleinman, Diane Kolyer, Geney Levin, Joanne Lipman, Gerry Logue, Karen Marcinczyk, Patrick McDonough, Cheryl McKenna, Sandi Mendelson, Jim Mezoff, Ivan Mogull, Susan Murcko, Gloria Neimark, Kathy O'Brien, Vanessa O'Connell, Aliah O'Neill and AIDS Walk NY, Neela Pal, Suzanne Sherman Propp, Iris Raylesberg, Amy Rhodes, Barbara Ross, Michael Rozansky, Ruth Sarfaty, Ava Seave, Ellen Ruth Seidman, Lauren Silva-Pinto, Carrie Sorensen, Carla Madeiros Starbuck, Jane Startz, Amanda Urban, Bonnie Verburg, Meredith Wagner, Stefanie Weiss, Nancy and Donald Wergeles, the Hyacinth Foundation, and the New Jersey Women and AIDS Network.

Thanks to Julie Mazur Tribe of Brooklyn Book Studio,

without whose expertise, wisdom, humanity, and patience there would be no book. Thank you also to Jennifer K. Beal Davis for her cover design and art direction, and Brett Miller for the layout.

Randi Clark, a celebrated professional horse photographer from Waco, Texas, found me online when seeking someone to talk to about the loss of her own husband. I'm so glad she did. Randi, thank you for not just being my friend, but also for the incredible support you've provided for this book. We walk in the same shoes, sister.

And to my Westport Book Group, among the smartest, most compassionate women I know, thank you for your steadfast encouragement and support every step of the way: Dr. Linda Gray, Jennifer Kanter, Marianna Kulak McCall, Lisa Mezoff, Maggie Mudd, Diana Muller, and Lauren Tarshis. "Angels in pajamas forever," ladies. (My dearest Mag, Lisa, and Marianna, thank you, again, for that memorable birthday drive to Brandywine, Pennsylvania, that started it all.)

Bill Kneip, my brother, you inspire me with your bravery and kindness. Keep the faith.

David Evans, I couldn't have made it without you.

Caroline and Daniel Andrew: for you I am grateful every single day.

About the Author

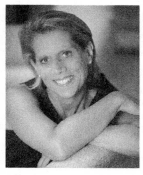

Photo by David Dreyfuss

MAGGIE KNEIP is a veteran of the publishing industry, with a career spanning more than two decades in publicity and marketing at Bertelsmann, Scholastic Inc., and Abrams Books. She has performed as a singer at such Manhattan clubs as the Laurie Beechman Theatre and the Metropolitan Room. Maggie graduated with degrees in English and theater from the College of William and Mary, and received a master of fine arts in dance from Sarah Lawrence College. Learn more about her at Maggiekneip.com, on Twitter at @magkneip, and on Facebook at facebook.com/noweveryonewillknow.

LAURA LANDRO (foreword) is an assistant managing editor for *The Wall Street Journal* and writes frequently on health care, including a column entitled "The Informed Patient." She is also the author of *Survivor: Taking Charge of Your Fight Against Cancer.*

DALE V. ATKINS, PHD (afterword), widely known as "Dr. Dale," is a licensed psychologist, popular keynote speaker, and author of six books and numerous chapters on social and relationship issues. She is a frequent commentator on NBC's *Today* show and CNN's *Headline News,* and has been an on-screen expert for several award-winning documentaries and news programs. She has a private psychology practice in New York City and can be found at www.drdaleatkins.com.

CPSIA information can be obtained at www.ICGtesting.com
Printed in the USA
BVOW08s1950021215

429186BV00005B/138/P